Oral Health and Heart Disease

BY
Sam Ziff
Michael F. Ziff, D.D.S.

Bio-Probe, Inc., Publisher
P.O. Box 608010 - Orlando, FL 32860-8010
(407) 290-9670 - FAX (407) 299-4149

This book is dedicated to providing the public and health professionals with scientific information related to periodontal disease and its effects on the heart. It is not intended as medical advice. Our intention is solely informational and educational. Please consult a Dentist, Physician or other Health Professional should the need for one be warranted.

Mention of trade names of products or companies does not constitute an endorsement of them by the authors or Bio-Probe, Inc. and is done solely for the purpose of providing relevant information to our readers.

© 2002 Bio-Probe, Inc.

All rights reserved.

No part of this book may be copied or reproduced in any form without written consent of the publisher.

ISBN 0-941011-17-8

Published in the United States of America

by Bio-Probe, Inc.

P.O. Box 608010 - Orlando, FL 32860-8010

(407) 290-9670 - FAX (407) 299-4149

Visit us on the Internet at http://www.bioprobe.com

Oral Health and Heart Disease

CONTENTS

Introduction 5
Chapter 1 Overview 7
Chapter 2 Periodontal disease and the risk of cardiovascular disease ... 13
Chapter 3 Other systemic diseases related to periodontal disease. 19
Chapter 4 Mercury and your heart 23
Chapter 5 Mercury damage to the heart and blood vessels. 31
Chapter 6 Things you can do. 43
Chapter 7 Nutritional support for a healthy mouth and heart. 55
Chapter 8 Biocompatible Periodontal Therapy (BPT) 77
Index 85

Oral Health and Heart Disease

Oral Health and Heart Disease

INTRODUCTION

In 1985 we wrote a book about the relationship of mercury to heart disease and how mercury from amalgam dental fillings maybe a hidden causal factor in the development of heart disease.

Since publication however, the world of science has exploded with information about systemic effects related to poor oral health from oral infections. Oral infections are capable of causing many different systemic health problems; however, because of the prior dental mercury/heart connection, and the fact that heart disease still remains the #1 cause of death, we are going to concentrate primarily on oral health problems as they relate to your heart.

Our purpose in revisiting the subject of the original book is to make information available to you the reader, that may change your life and reduce or eliminate the potential for a serious cardiac event.

We are providing information on the following areas, all related directly or indirectly to oral health:
- Periodontal disease and its relationship to the heart.
- Plaque and tartar as a source of bacteria
- Amalgam dental fillings as a cause of periodontal disease.
- Bacteremia from the oral cavity.
- Root canals as a source of bacteremia.
- Mercury and your heart.
- Mercury and its effect on your nutritional status of key nutrients involved in the maintenance of a healthy heart.
- Nutritional support for a healthy mouth and heart
- What is wrong with the current philosophies on treating periodontal disease.
- The International Academy of Oral Medicine and Toxicology (IAOMT) protocol for treating periodontal disease.

Oral Health and Heart Disease

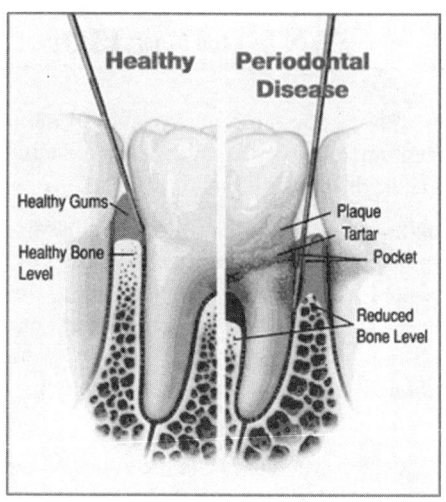

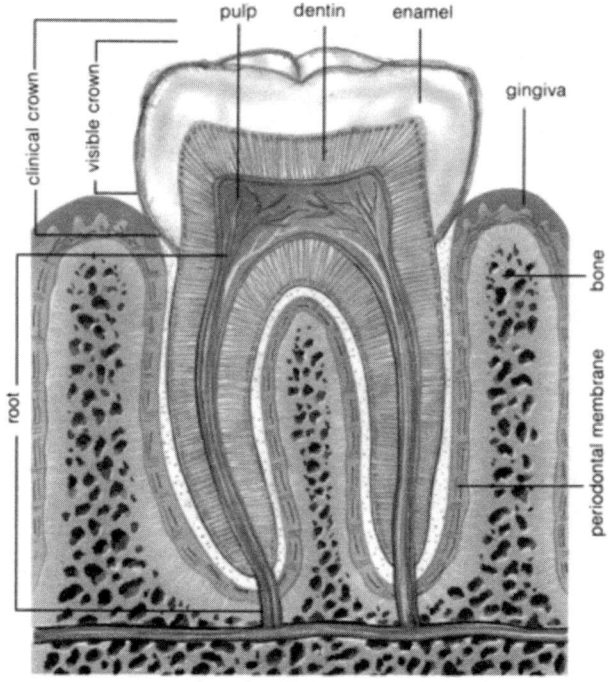

CHAPTER 1

The Overview

Cardiovascular diseases as a whole represent the No. 1 cause of death in the United States, accounting for 950,000 deaths annually (about 41 percent of total mortality from all causes). Coronary Heart Disease (CHD) by itself accounts for about 460,000 deaths annually.(1)

An important point to be made here is that although death rates from cardiovascular diseases have been declining over the past decades it is not because there are fewer cardiovascular events happening. The decline is due to improved survival of patients experiencing clinical events.(2) So, although fewer people are dying after experiencing a cardiovascular event, overall the number of events occurring annually has not declined and in fact, may have increased.

Over the years, the medical profession has identified the following risk factors for heart disease:

Cigarette Smoking,

High Blood Cholesterol Levels,

High Blood Pressure,

Physical Inactivity,

Diabetes,,

Stress,

Obesity.

Despite improved clinical care, heightened public awareness, and widespread use of health innovations, coronary heart disease (CHD) remains the leading cause of death in the United States, and the decline in rates from CHD that began during the 1960s slowed during the 1990s. During 2001, approximately 1.1 million persons are expected to have a CHD event. Prevention remains the key strategy for reducing CHD mortality.(3)

An estimated 12 million persons in the United States have CHD. Of the 1.1 million persons who are expected to have a CHD event during 2001, approximately 650,000 will be first events and 450,000 will be recurrences. Each year,

Oral Health and Heart Disease

approximately 220,000 fatal CHD events occur suddenly among unhospitalized persons. The slowing decline in CHD death rates may be explained by the pattern of CHD risk factors reported during the 1990s. Minimal, if any, improvement has occurred in preventive behaviors (e.g., adequate physical activity, cessation of smoking, and the control of high blood pressure).(3)

Hundreds of millions of dollars have been spent advertising all of the established risk factors and providing education programs and literature to the American people. However, as stated above by the Centers For Disease Control (CDC) these efforts have not had a major impact or provided any reduction of cardiovascular disease. It would appear reasonable then to believe that the authorities have overlooked some other factors that must have equal or greater significance than all the other identified risk factors.

We believe that oral health is a major factor in cardiac health that has been totally ignored until very recently. These recent studies have primarily focused on the discovery that bacteria related to periodontal disease have been found in the heart and other organs. Thus, providing proof that oral bacteria can and do in fact travel systemically all over the body. Most researchers are now including periodontal disease as another risk factor.

The most common dental filling material over the last hundred years has been "silver/amalgam." Whatever the reasons or motives behind it, the use of the word silver to describe this type of filling is a misnomer. The correct designation should be mercury dental fillings, as mercury comprises 50% or more of the material actually used to fill the cavity in the tooth. However, for clarity in presentation we will call them amalgam dental fillings, as there are several metals that comprise amalgam: mercury, silver, copper, zinc. This aspect is important because allergic reactions have been reported for all of the metals contained in amalgam dental fillings.

Speaking of allergic reactions, it is important to note that the American Dental Association (ADA) as well as the Food and Drug Administration (FDA) and the National Institute of Dental and Craniofacial Research (NIDCR) feel that amalgam dental fillings are safe except in those few individual who may be allergic to them. However, this position flies in the face of overwhelming scientific data demonstrating the opposite. The most recent of these studies involved 2300-2600 patients who were allergy tested with a dental screening series. The results are pretty startling in that 13% reacted to ammoniated mercury and 10.3% reacted to mercury.(4) Nobody knows exactly how many individuals in the United States

Oral Health and Heart Disease

have amalgam dental fillings. We feel a conservative estimate wo. 125 million with one or more amalgam dental fillings. 10.3% of 1z. means that almost 13 million people have an allergy to the mercury i. amalgam dental fillings and in most instances, they and their physician have no idea that their fillings might be causing whatever reactivity they are displaying or experiencing

The basic problem with amalgam dental fillings is that they are unstable and that their mercury content is continuously out-gassing or leaking out of the fillings in the form of mercury vapor which you are continually inhaling into your lungs, where 80-100% is absorbed into your blood. Inhaled mercury vapor remains in its vapor form through about four complete circulations of your blood where, as a vapor, it readily passes the blood-brain barrier and enters the brain, heart, and every important organ in the body. To put the average amount of mercury contained in one amalgam filling in perspective, there is enough mercury in one large filling to contaminate a 10 square mile lake sufficiently to restrict fishing.

Mercury is one the most toxic metals on earth and its use as a dental material in the year 2001 is unconscionable. However, we will discuss the dangers of mercury in subsequent chapters. At this time it is important to point out that one aspect of having amalgam dental fillings that is not talked about by the dental profession is that they can and do cause periodontal problems.

The following information dealing with amalgam dental fillings and periodontal disease has been taken from a presentation made by Michael F. Ziff, D.D.S. at a 1991 National Institute of Health Technology Assessment Conference.(5)

The first formal investigation of the effect of amalgam fillings on the periodontal structure was done by Zander in 1957. Clinical and histologic examination confirmed inflammatory response in gingival tissue adjacent to amalgam fillings. These findings were subsequently confirmed and expanded upon over the years by many different studies. Most researchers found that the tissue response to mercury was the same as the tissue response to calculus or tartar as it is commonly called. Consequently, amalgam fillings should be considered a causal factor in the development of periodontal disease the same as tartar. Just so there is no mistake in anyone's mind, the development of periodontal disease in tissues touching amalgam fillings, is not just because of irritation of the tissue. A Study done in 1974 analyzed biopsies of tissues that were in contact with amalgam fillings and found markedly higher mercury content than did the control biopsies. A 1976 study demonstrated that the normal corrosion products from amalgam

Oral Health and Heart Disease

fillings, which contained mercury, silver, copper and zinc ions, produced injurious (cytotoxic) effects on human gingival fibroblasts in vitro.(5)

It doesn't take a great stretch of ones imagination to visualize why the rate of periodontal disease is 35% or more(6), when it is estimated that there are more than 125 million Americans with amalgam dental fillings. Although suitable and biocompatible dental materials have been available for years, amalgam fillings are still being implanted into the teeth of unsuspecting and uniformed patients at the rate of 75 million plus each year.

The fact that amalgam dental fillings can cause periodontal disease coupled with the fact that bacteria from periodontal disease transfer systemically to the heart and other organs is not a condition conducive to good health.

Oral Health and Heart Disease

REFERENCES:

1. 2001 Heart and Stroke Statistical Update. American Heart Association.
2. Schmermund A, Erbel R. Med Klin 2001 May 15;96(5):261-269. (Article in German)
3. Mortality From Coronary Heart Disease and Acute Myocardial Infarction United States, 1998. *MMWR* 50(06):90-93, Centers For Disease Control.
4. Kanerva L., et al. A Multicenter study of patch test reactions with dental screening series. Am J Contact Dermatitis; 2001 Jun;12(2):83-87.
5. Ziff MF. Documented Clinical Side-effects to Dental Amalgam. Advances in Dental Research. Effects and Side-Effects of Dental Restorative Materials. IADR Sept 1992, Vol 6:131-134.
6. Albandar JM, Brunelle JA, Kingman A. Destructive periodontal disease in adults 30 years of age and older in the United States, 1984-1988. J Periodontol. 1999 Jan;70(1):13-29.

Oral Health and Heart Disease

CHAPTER 2

PERIODONTAL DISEASE AND THE RISK OF CARDIOVASCULAR DISEASE

We would like to start this Chapter with a definition of the word "metastasis." Traditionally, people only associate the word metastasis with cancer. Consequently, we feel it is important for everyone to understand the broader meaning of metastasis:

"The transfer of disease from one organ or part to another not directly connected with it. It may be due either to the transfer of pathogenic microorganisms (e.g., tubercle bacilli) or to transfer of cells, as in malignant tumors."(Dorland's Medical Dictionary) This definition has a bearing on the information that follows.

Periodontal diseases, (including gingivitis and periodontitis) are serious infections that, left untreated, can lead to tooth loss. The word periodontal literally means "around the tooth." Periodontitis disease is a chronic infection that effects the gums and bone supporting the teeth.

Periodontal disease can affect one tooth or many teeth. It begins when the bacteria in plaque (the sticky, colorless film that constantly forms on your teeth) causes the gums to become inflamed.

In the mildest form of the disease, gingivitis, the gums redden, swell and bleed easily. There is usually little or no discomfort. Gingivitis is often caused by inadequate oral hygiene. Gingivitis is reversible with professional treatment and good oral home care.

Untreated gingivitis can advance to periodontitis. With time, plaque can spread and grow below the gum line. Toxins produced by the bacteria in plaque irritate the gums. The toxins stimulate a chronic inflammatory response in which the body in essence turns on itself, and the tissues and bone that support the teeth are broken down and destroyed. Gums separate from the teeth, forming pockets (spaces between the teeth and gums) that become infected. As the disease progresses, the pockets deepen and more gum tissue and bone are destroyed. Often, this destructive process has very mild symptoms. Eventually, teeth can become loose and have to be removed.. (The above descriptions were taken from

Oral Health and Heart Disease

The American Academy of Periodontology web page; http://www.perio.org/consumer/2a.html)

The warning signs of the disease are a bad taste in the mouth, bad breath, red or swollen gums, tender gums, bleeding gums, loose teeth, sensitive teeth, pain when chewing, pus around teeth and gums, and brown, hard deposits, called calculus on the surface of the teeth. The best treatment for gingivitis is prevention with good oral hygiene.

Traditionally, the major concern of the medical and dental professions regarding dental work and heart disease has primarily been "infective endocarditis" (IE). IE is a serious disease involving the membrane lining the chambers of the heart; the immediate concern of the medical profession appears to be preventing bacterial growth on the heart valves. The standard dental protocol is that if you are going to work on a patient that has certain heart problems, you have to utilize antibiotics to minimize systemic bacterial transfer related to any dental procedure contemplated.

The most common dental diseases, periodontal disease and dental caries, are chronic infections caused by bacteria of normal oral flora. **When these bacteria increase in number and irritation and exceed the host defense threshold, disease arises.** Human endodontic and periodontal infections are associated with complex microfloras in which approximately 150, (in apical periodontitis) and 350 (in marginal periodontitis) bacterial species have been encountered. A variety of clinical procedures can cause the translocation of microorganisms from the oral cavity to the bloodstream.(1)

Recent research studying possible relationships between periodontal disease and heart disease have been greatly expanded beyond that of infective endocarditis. It is now scientifically established that periodontal disease is a potential risk factor for coronary heart disease. A very recent study now expands this risk to cerebrovascular accidents (CVAs). The study used 9962 adults aged 25-74 who participated in the First National Health and Nutrition Examination Survey (NHANES I) and its follow-up study and after evaluation of all the data concluded that: "Periodontal disease is an important risk factor for total CVA and, in particular, nonhemorrhagic stroke."(2)

In 1989 a group of Finnish investigators associated dental infections with cerebral and acute myocardial infarctions. The authors took into consideration for their statistical analysis **all of the common risk factors for stroke and heart attack,**

Oral Health and Heart Disease

including age, smoking, high levels of serum lipids, diabetes and socioeconomic status. Accounting for all of these factors, however, **did not eliminate the statistically significant association between oral infections and cardiovascular disease.**(3-4)

A recent study published in December 2000, provided further confirmation of the Finnish study. The authors concluded that the results of their study indicated that periodontal disease may be associated with acute myocardial infarction.(5)

Additionally, several studies have now concluded that there is a relationship between systemic bacteria from periodontal disease and the development of atherosclerosis. Periodontal pathogens are present in atherosclerotic plaques where, like other infectious microorganisms such as Chlamydia pneumoniae, they may play a role in the development and progression of atherosclerosis leading to coronary vascular disease and other clinical problems.(6)

BACTEREMIA

Bacteremia is defined as "the presence of bacteria in the blood." Although infections of the skin or any part of the body can cause bacteremia, there are several bacteria that are only, or primarily found in the mouth. Researchers have determined that almost any procedure performed in the mouth can cause some degree of bacteremia. Transient bacteremia can occur for years in patients with chronic oral infections such as periodontal disease. Bacteria has been found in the blood after tooth-brushing (40 percent of the subjects), tooth extraction (60 percent) and periodontal surgery (88 percent).(7) This includes even having orthodontic bands placed or taken off. This situation is greatly aggravated if there is any type of inflammation or infection such as in periodontal disease or gingivitis. Procedures involved in hygienists or dentists cleaning your teeth and scaling below the gum line are especially troublesome because of the increased potential of causing bacteremia.

Thrombo-embolic (clotting-blockage) complications including stroke and myocardial infarction are common in bacteremic patients with and without endocarditis: about 20% of patients with infective endocarditis will develop stroke during their disease. About 10% of bacteremic patients without endocarditis will develop stroke within one month of the onset of bacteremia and about 4% of bacteremic patients will develop myocardial infarction. It has been estimated that

Oral Health and Heart Disease

about 10% of all strokes are associated with bacteremic infections.(8) Those are extremely powerful statistics.

At the recent World Congress of Neurology 18-22 June 2001, Ruth Bonita of the World Health Organization (WHO) made a prediction that by the year 2020, stroke will be the leading cause of death and disability, accounting for between 7 and 10 million deaths per year worldwide, or 12 strokes per second.(9) Missing from all the discussions and presentations of the participants about actions that could be taken to address this problem, no mention was made of an association between periodontal disease and stroke. It is a tragedy that the world scientists in neurology are not aware of or, addressing the benefits to humankind that would accrue from world-wide implementation of sound oral hygiene practices and the total elimination of amalgam dental fillings.

Consequently, taken as a whole, you as an individual, have to realize that oral health means much more than just cursorily brushing your teeth once or twice a day.

ROOT CANALS AS A SOURCE OF BACTEREMIA

It has been established that apical periodontitis with bone resorption cannot develop in the absence of bacteria in the root canal system.(10) In a recent investigation designed to determine if endodontically treated teeth do cause bacteremia, microbiological samples were taken from the root canals of 26 patients with asymptomatic apical periodontitis of single-rooted teeth. The blood of the patients was drawn during and 10 minutes after endodontic therapy. The patients blood was then analyzed for the presence of bacteria. All root canals contained anaerobic bacteria. The frequency of bacteremia varied from 31% to 54%. The microorganisms from the root canal and blood presented identical phenotype and genetic characteristics with the patients examined, demonstrating that endodontic treatment can be the cause of anaerobic bacteremia.(11)

In a more recent study, done in the year 2000, DNA-DNA hybridization techniques were used to identify bacteria in periapical endodontic lesions of asymptomatic teeth. Bacterial DNA was identified in all samples taken from the 34 patients involved in the study. This study provided solid evidence that bacteria invade the periapical tissue of asymptomatic teeth with apical periodontitis.(12)

In this study, a total of 1001 endodontically treated teeth were evaluated independently by two examiners to determine the success rate of the treatment. The success rate for all endodontically treated teeth was 67.4%. This means that failures comprised 32.6%, which is vastly larger than previous estimates of a routine 10% failure rate in endodontically treated teeth. This particular study only evaluated the technical quality of the root filling and the technical quality of the coronal restoration.(13) It did not address bacterial infection and inflammation which are usually the two consequences of root canal failure.

There is another aspect of root canal infections that bears on your ability to control the infection satisfactorily. That is bacteria can develop resistance to antibiotics complicating the medical job of treating the infection.

OCCLUSION AND PROGRESSION OF PERIODONTITIS

Occlusion in simple terms is when the teeth in the upper and lower jaws are able to provide the highest efficiency in chewing without producing any trauma. It has previously been hypothesized that malocclusion could increase the severity of periodontal disease. However, there has not been much research on this until recently. An April 2001 study has now provided strong evidence of an association between untreated occlusal discrepancies and the progression of periodontal disease. Perhaps more importantly, the study showed that occlusal treatment significantly reduced the progression of periodontal disease over time and can be an important adjunct therapy in the comprehensive treatment of periodontal disease.(14)

Oral Health and Heart Disease

REFERENCES:

1. Debelian GJ, Olsen I, Tronstad L. Systemic diseases caused by oral microorganissms. Endod Dent Traumatol 1994 Apr;10(2):57-65.

2. Wu T, et al. Periodontal disease and risk of cerebrovascular disease: the first national health and nutrition examination survey and its follow-up study. Arch Inter Med 2000 Oct 9;160(18):2749-2755.

3. Syrjanen J, et al. Dental infections in association with cerebral infarction in young and middle-aged men. J Inter Med 1989;25:179-184.

4. Mattila KJ, Nieminen MS, Valtonen V, et al. Association between dental health and acute myocardial infarction. Br Med J 1989;3(1):206-211.

5. Emingil G., et al. Association between periodontal disease and acute myocardial infarction. J Periodontol 2000 Dec;71(12):1882-1886.

6. Haraszthy VI, et al. Identification of periodontal pathogens in atheromatous plaques. Periodontol 2000 Oct;71(10):1554-1560.

7. Herzberg MC, Meyer MW. Effects of oral flora on platelets: possible consequences in cardiovascular disease. Periodontol 1996;67(supple 10):1138-1142.

8. Valtonen V, Kuikka A, Syrjanen J. Thrombo-embolic complications in bacteraemic infections. Eur Heart J. 1995 Dec;14 Suppl K:20-23.

9. World Congress of Neurology 2001: Diseases of old age threaten to dominate populations by Julie Clayton, 22 June 2001. BioMedNet News and Comment.

10. Tronstad L. Recent developments in endodontic research. Scand J Dent Res 1992 Feb;100(1):52-59.

11. Debelian GJ, Olsen I, Tronstad L. Anaerobic bacteremia and fungemia in patients undergoing endodontic therapy: an overview. Ann Periodontol 1998.Jul;3(1):281-287.

12. Sunde PT, Tronstad L, Eribe ER, Lindo PO, Olsen I. Assessment of periradicular microbiota by DNA-DNA hybridization. Endod Dent Traumatol 2000 Oct;16(5):191-196.

13. Tronstad L, Asbjornsen K, Doving L, Pedersen I, Eriksen HM. Influence of coronal restorations on the periapical health of endodontically treated teeh. Endod Dent Traumatol 2000 Oct;16(5):218-221.

14. Harrel SK, Nunn ME. The effect of occlusal discrepancies on periodontitis. II. Relationship of occlusal treatment to the progression of periodontal disease. J Periodontol 2001 Apr;72(4):495-505.

CHAPTER 3

OTHER SYSTEMIC DISEASES RELATED TO PERIODONTAL DISEASE

The information provided in this chapter is intended only to demonstrate the scope of the effect of poor oral health and its impact on development or exacerbation of other serious health problems. It is apparent to us from the scientific research to date, that future research will show causal relationships between oral health and other diseases or syndromes. However, heart disease remains the primary focus of this book.

LOW BIRTH WEIGHT

Pregnancy can influence oral health. Hormonal changes during pregnancy can promote inflamed gingiva without changes in the plaque level.(1-2) Birth control pills may also cause inflammation of the gingiva without necessarily increasing the plaque level.(3)

Several studies have now concluded that periodontal disease represents a clinically significant risk factor for preterm low birth weight as a consequence of either preterm labor (less than 37 weeks) or premature rupture of membranes.(4-5) The incidence of low birth weight and preterm delivery remains at about 10% of all live births in the United States.(6)

In preterm infants low birth weight remains a significant cause of perinatal (the period occurring shortly before and after birth) morbidity (increased prevalence of disease) and mortality.(7)

DIABETES AND PERIODONTAL DISEASE

Several studies have been done on the relationship between periodontal disease and diabetes. Some studies are suggesting that this relationship goes both ways - periodontal disease may make it more difficult for people who have diabetes to control their blood sugar and conversely, diabetes is a risk factor for severe periodontal disease.(8)

Oral Health and Heart Disease

In another study dealing with patients with insulin-dependent diabetes mellitus (IDDM) the authors stated that they thought their study suggested that hyperglycemia could indirectly exacerbate inflammatory tissue destruction through the body's scavenger system against advanced glycation end products, and that both hyper- and hypoglycemia might directly impair the biological function of periodontal connective tissues through cell-matrix interactions. (9)

A longitudinal study of diabetes and periodontal disease has been carried out in the Pima tribe, an Indian population in the United States having a prevalence of non-insulin dependent diabetes of about 50%, the highest reported prevalence in the world.(10-11). The study results indicated that severe periodontitis at baseline is associated with increased risk of poor glycemic control at follow-up two or more years later. These findings suggest that severe periodontitis may be an important risk factor in the progression of diabetes, and control of periodontal infections is essential to achieve long-term control of diabetes mellitus.

Is this relationship between oral health and diabetes important? Diabetes mellitus affects more than 12 million people in the United States, and is characterized by metabolic abnormalities and long -term complications involving the eyes, kidneys, nervous system, vasculature and periodontium.(12)

POOR ORAL HEALTH AND CHRONIC LUNG DISEASE

Recent studies utilizing data from the third National Health and Nutrition Examination Survey (NHANES III) have demonstrated a relationship between oral health and lung diseases. One aspect involves "aspirating pneumonia" (pneumonia due to the entrance food or other foreign matter into the respiratory passages). "Pneumonia can result from infection by anaerobic bacteria. Dental plaque would seem to be a logical source of these bacteria, especially in patients with periodontal disease. Such patients harbor a large number of subgingival bacteria, particularly anaerobic species."(12)

Limeback (13) noted a relationship between poor oral hygiene and aspiration pneumonia among elderly residents of chronic care facilities. He subsequently found that the nursing homes with the least number of dental visits had the most deaths due to pneumonia.

In another study using the NHANES III data, individuals with either chronic bronchitis and/or emphysema, together considered as chronic obstructive pulmonary disease (COPD) were evaluated for lung function and oral health. Subjects

Oral Health and Heart Disease

with a history of COPD had more periodontal attachment loss than subjects without COPD. Subjects with a mean attachment loss greater than 3.0 mm had a higher risk of COPD than those having less than 3.0 mm. A trend was noted in that lung function appeared to diminish with increasing periodontal attachment loss.(14)

Oral Health and Heart Disease

REFERENCES:

1. Loe H and Silness J. Periodontal disease in pregnancy: prevalence and severity. Acta Odontol Scand 1963 21:532-551.
2. Kornman KS, Loesche WJ. The subgingival microbial flora during pregnancy J Periodontal Res 1980 Mar;15(2):111-122.
3. Kalkwarf KL. Effect of oral contraceptive therapy on gingival inflammation in humans. J Periodontol 1978 Nov;49(11):560-563.
4. Offenbacher S., et al. Periodontal infection as a possible risk factor for preterm low birth weight. J Periodontol 1996 Oct;67(10 Suppl):103-113.
5. Offenbacher S, Beck JD, Lieff S, Slade G. Role of periodontitis in systemic health: spontaneous preterm birth. J Dent Educ 1998 Oct;62(10):852-858.
6. Davenport ES., et al. The East London Study of maternal chronic periodontal disease and preterm low birth weight infants: study design and prevalence data. Ann Periodontol 1998 Jul;3(1):213-221.
7. McCormick MC The contribution of low birth weight to infant mortality and childhood morbidity. N Engl J Med 1985 Jan 10;312(2):82-90.
8. Grossi SG, Genco RJ. Periodontal disease and diabetes mellitus: a two-way relationship. Ann Periodontol 1998 Jul;3(1):51-61.
9. Nishimura F., et al. Periodontal disease as a complication of diabetes mellitus. Ann Periodontol 1998 Jul;3(1):20-29.
10. Shlossman M., et al. Type 2 diabetes mellitus and periodontal disease. J Am Dent Assoc 1990 Oct;121(4):532-536.
11. Knowler WC, Pettitt DJ, Saad MF, Bennett PH. Diabetes mellitus in the Pima Indians: Incidence, risk factors and pathogenesis. Diabetes Metab Rev. 1990 Feb;6(1):1-27.
12. Li X, Kristin M, Kolltveit KM, Tronstad L, Olsen I. Systemic diseases caused by oral infection. Clin Microbiol Rev 2000 Oct;13(4):547-558.
13. Limeback H. The relationshp between oral health and systemic infections among elderly residents of chronic care facilities. Gerodontology 1998;7:131-137.
14. Scannapieco FA, Ho AW. Potential associations between chronic respiratory disease and periodontal disease: analysis of National Health and Nutrition Examination Survey III. J Periodontol 2001 Jan;72(1):50-56.

CHAPTER 4
MERCURY AND YOUR HEART

Published animal studies and human autopsy studies have scientifically confirmed, without a shadow of doubt, that people with dental amalgam fillings are constantly absorbing mercury from these fillings. Animal studies performed in the 1960's and early 1970's established that exposure to mercury, especially mercury vapor, resulted in mercury accumulation in the brain. This is why human autopsy studies on dental amalgam subjects have concentrated on measuring mercury accumulations in the brain. Little attention was paid to mercury accumulation in the heart, though historically, as is discussed in the next chapter, mercury exposure has been shown to have a harmful affect on the heart. Medical scientific researchers began investigating mercury accumulations in cardiovascular tissue of humans and animals in controlled experiments in the 1950's.

NON-DENTAL MERCURY IN CARDIOVASCULAR TISSUES

In 1954, C.G. Griffin and associates investigated the presence of a number of metals in various human tissues. The heart tissue of 45 subjects was analyzed for mercury content and was found to average 0.27 milligrams of mercury per 100 grams dry tissue. These subjects had been given mercury diuretics as treatment for congestive heart failure.

In 1970 and 1971, researchers at Washington University School of Medicine in St. Louis, Missouri injected inorganic mercury into animals and measured the levels of mercury in blood and various tissues. The highest levels of mercury, other than those found in the kidney, were in the aorta tissue. Significant levels of mercury were also found in the heart tissue.

In 1983, G.F. Placidi and his associates exposed animals to radioactively labeled mercury vapor by inhalation. Utilizing whole-body autoradiogram, they found a significant uptake of mercury by the kidney, brain, heart muscle, intestine and liver in decreasing order.

It has also been shown in animal studies that exposure to mercury vapor results in much larger accumulations of mercury in the heart than does exposure to inorganic mercury. In an animal study on mice, published in 1983, Khayat and

Oral Health and Heart Disease

Dencker compared mercury accumulations in the heart and other tissues from equal exposures to radioactive inhaled mercury vapor and injected mercuric chloride (inorganic mercury). The animals exposed to mercury vapor had much higher levels of mercury in the heart and brain, as well as larger amounts in the thyroid, adrenals, spinal ganglia and nerves, testes, and ovaries.

In 1984, Khayat and Dencker set out to determine if other animals showed the same patterns as did the mice. They performed another study of the distribution of inhaled mercury vapor, this time using monkeys and rats. Once again, they found high accumulations of mercury in the heart tissues of animals exposed to inhaled radioactive mercury vapor. The mercury levels in the heart were three to four times those found in the brain of exposed animals, after only one hour of exposure. The authors concluded that in mice, rats and monkeys the lungs, brain, and heart all accumulate mercury after exposure to inhaled mercury vapor, indicating that these are target organs in most species, including humans.

In 1989, M. Yoshida and associates exposed newborn guinea pigs and their mothers to mercury vapor and measured the amounts of mercury in blood and various tissues directly after exposure. Mercury levels were much higher in the blood, brain, lungs, and heart tissue of the newborn babies than in the mothers. The mercury levels in the heart tissue of the newborn babies was two and a half to five times higher than levels in the brain tissue.

Also in 1989, Carmignani and associates exposed rats to inorganic mercury in drinking water for 350 days and compared the tissue levels of mercury to control animals that had received pure water during that same time. The levels of mercury found in the heart tissue of exposed rats was 60% of the levels found in brain tissue, and about twenty times the level found in the heart tissue of control animals.

In the same year (1989) Japanese researchers (Matsuo and associates) investigated mercury levels in the heart tissue of adults. Levels of inorganic mercury, methylmercury, and total mercury were determined in 46 subjects. Significantly high levels of mercury were found in heart tissue, about the same amounts as were found in the brain. It was also found that the levels of inorganic mercury in the heart increased with age, while the levels of methylmercury decreased. The authors noted that people are chronically exposed to mercury vapor from dental amalgam fillings.

Oral Health and Heart Disease

A recent (1999) study done by Frustaci and colleagues from the Cardiology, Catholic University, in Rome Italy, investigated the pos. genic role of trace element levels in the muscular tissue of the heart (my Biopsy samples from 13 patients with clinical hemodynamic and his ogy diagnosis of idiopathic dilated cardiomyopathy (IDCM) were analyzed by neutron activation analysis for 32 different trace elements. (The definition of "dilated cardiomyopathy" is: A syndrome of ventricular dilation, systolic contractile dysfunction, and, often, congestive heart failure; the course is usually progressive with poor prognosis. It is believed to be an expression of heart muscle damage caused by a variety of factors. Idiopathic is defined as self-originated; or of unknown cause.)

In patients with IDCM the mean mercury concentration was 22,000 times (178,400 ng/g vs. 8 ng/g), antimony 12,000 times, gold 11 times, chromium 13 times, and cobalt 4 times higher than in control subjects. The researchers concluded that the increased concentration of trace elements in patients with IDCM may adversely effect mitochondria activity and myocardial metabolism and worsen cellular function.

RESEARCH IN ANIMALS AND HUMANS HAS PROVEN THAT MERCURY BUILDS UP IN HEART TISSUE AND IN BLOOD VESSELS AND THAT EXPOSURE TO MERCURY VAPOR CAUSES THE GREATEST ACCUMULATION!

DENTAL AMALGAM MERCURY IN BODY TISSUES

Now that it has been scientifically confirmed that mercury exits dental amalgam fillings, researchers have been turning their attention to determining if this mercury enters body tissues and, if so, the specific organs and tissues in which this mercury accumulates.

In his human autopsy studies, Dr. Magnus Nylander in Sweden found high levels of mercury in the pituitary glands of dental personnel and in subjects with amalgams. A research team in Canada, led by Drs. Murray Vimy and Fritz Lorscheider, placed amalgam fillings in the teeth of pregnant sheep. Within days they found mercury within the bodies of the unborn babies. Meanwhile, the same research team is tracing the amalgam-derived mercury into specific body tissues. This team has now confirmed these findings in the monkey, which is a primate with physiologic characteristics very similar to humans.

Oral Health and Heart Disease

This experiment dramatically demonstrates that mercury absorbed amalgam is rapidly taken up by the heart tissue, in even greater amount rapidly than that which is absorbed into the brain. Although the dental amalgam was not implanted into the teeth and left there to release mercury during use, other animal studies, as well as the three human autopsy studies, have proven that mercury from dental amalgams placed in teeth is absorbed into the brain tissue.

In 1987, Dr. Bengt Fredin doing research in Sweden, implanted mercury amalgam fillings into the teeth of guinea pigs and sacrificed the animals at periods of one day, three days, five days, and ten days. He measured the amount of mercury in the brain, heart, liver, kidney, blood, and urine and compared them to control animals who did not have mercury amalgam fillings. After one day, the mercury levels in the heart averaged ten times that found in brain tissue; after three days, the heart mercury levels were three and a half to ten times that in the brain; after five days it was almost twice the brain mercury levels; and at ten days the amount of mercury in the heart was still 50% more than that found in the brain. This animal study confirmed that inhaled mercury vapor from dental amalgam rapidly accumulated in the heart tissue more so than in the brain. It also established that the source of mercury in the heart tissue could be dental amalgam fillings in function, i.e. mercury released from chewing.

IN ANIMALS, MERCURY VAPOR RELEASED FROM DENTAL AMALGAM FILLINGS IN FUNCTION ACCUMULATED MORE RAPIDLY IN HEART TISSUE THAN IN THE BRAIN!

The research team at the University of Calgary School of Medicine, led by Drs. Murray J. Vimy and Fritz Lorscheider, utilized sheep as the experimental model. By incorporating a portion of radioactively labeled mercury into the amalgam fillings, they could trace mercury specifically from the dental amalgam into body tissues.

Within days after placement of the amalgam fillings in mothers, amalgam-derived mercury was found in the heart tissue of both mothers and unborn babies. The levels of mercury found in the heart tissues were comparable to levels found in the brain tissue of the animals. It is also interesting to note that the researchers found extremely high levels of amalgam-derived mercury in the pituitary glands of the unborn babies.

Oral Health and Heart Disease

Siblerud, in a 1990 human study comparing subjects with and without amalgam, showed that amalgam-bearing subjects had significantly higher blood pressure, lower heart rate, lower hemoglobin, and lower hematocrit. Hemoglobin, hematocrit, and red blood cells were significantly lower when correlated to increased levels of urine mercury. The subjects with amalgam dental fillings had a greater incidence of chest pains, tachycardia, anemia, fatigue, tiring easily, and being tired in the morning. The data suggest that inorganic mercury poisoning from dental amalgam does effect the cardiovascular system.

MERCURY DERIVED FROM DENTAL AMALGAM FILLINGS IN FUNCTION HAS BEEN TRACED DIRECTLY TO THE HEART TISSUES!

SUMMARY

Scientifically, more than sufficient evidence indicates that the heart is indeed a target organ for exposure to mercury, especially mercury vapor. It has now been firmly established that mercury specifically derived from dental amalgam fillings rapidly accumulates in the heart tissue. It must also be remembered that the brain, pituitary, thyroid, and adrenals also influence heart function and are also target organs after exposure to mercury vapor. Hopefully, researchers will soon begin investigating direct correlations between heart disease and the presence of mercury-releasing dental amalgam fillings. In the next chapter we will discuss the documented research demonstrating that mercury exposure does result in cardiovascular pathology.

Oral Health and Heart Disease

REFERENCES:

- Cutright, DE. et al. Systemic Mercury Levels Caused by Inhaling Mist During High-speed Amalgam Grinding. J oral Med. 28(4):100-4. October-December 1973.
- Carmignani, M. et al. Renal Ultrastructural Alterations and Cardiovascular Functional Changes in Rats Exposed to Mercuric Chloride. Arch Toxicol. Suppl 13:353-6. 1989.
- Danscher, G. et al. Traces of Mercury in Organs from Primates with Amalgam Fillings. Exper Molec Pathology. 52:291-9. 1990.
- Fredin, B. The Distribution of Mercury in Various Tissues of Guinea Pigs After Application of Dental Amalgam Fillings (A Pilot Study). Sci Total Environ. 66:263-8. 1987.
- Frustaci A., et al. Marked elevation of myocardial trace elements in idiopathic dilated cardiomyopathy compared with secondary cardiac dysfunction. J Am Coll Cardiol 1999 May;33(6):1578-1583.
- Griffith, CG. et al. The Inorganic Element Content of Certain Human Tissues. Ann Internal Med. 41:501-9. 1954.
- Hahn, LJ; Kloiber, R; Vimy, MJ; Takahashi, Y; Lorscheider, FL. Dental "Silver" Fillings: A Source of Mercury Exposure Revealed by Whole-body Image Scan and Tissue Analysis. FASEB J. 3:641-6. Dec 1989.
- Hahn, LJ; Kloiber, R; Leininger, RW; Vimy, MJ; Lorscheider, FL. Whole-body Imaging of the Distribution of Mercury Released from Dental Fillings into Monkey Tissues. FASEB J. 4:3256-60. Nov 1990.
- Khayat, A. & Dencker, L. Whole Body and Liver Distribution of Inhaled Mercury Vapor in the Mouse: Influence of Ethanol and Aminothiazole Pretreatment. J Appl Toxicol. 3(2):66-73. 1983.
- Khayat, A. & Dencker, L. Organ and Cellular Distribution of Inhaled Metallic Mercury in the Rat and Marmoset Monkey (Callithrix Jacchus): Influence of Ethyl Alcohol Pretreatment. Acta Pharmacol et Toxicol. 55:145-52. 1984.
- Matsuo, N; Suzuki, T; Akagi, H. Mercury Concentrations in Organs of Contemporary Japanese. Arch Environ Health. 44(5):298-303. Sept-Oct 1989.
- Nylander, M. Mercury in the Pituitary Glands of Dentists. Lancet. Pg. 442. Feb 22, 1986.
- Perry, HM, Jr.; Erlanger, M; Yunice, A; Schoepfle, E; Perry, EF. Hypertension and Tissue Metal Levels Following Intravenous Cadmium, Mercury, and Zinc. Amer J Physiol. 219:755-61. Sep 1970.
- Perry, HM, Jr.; Erlanger, M. Hypertension and Tissue Metal Levels After Intraperitoneal Cadmium, Mercury, and Zinc. Amer J Physiol. 220:808-11. March 1971.
- Placidi, GF; Dell'Osso, L; Viola, PL; Bertelli, A. Distribution of Inhaled Mercury (203 Hg) in Various Organs. Int J Tiss React. 5:193-200. 1983.
- Siblerud RI. The relationship between mercury from dental amalgam and the cardiovascular system. Sci Total Environ 1990 Dec 1;99(1-2):22-35.

Oral Health and Heart Disease

- Vimy, MJ; Takahashi, Y; Lorscheider, FL. Maternal-fetal Distribution of mercury (203 Hg) Released From Dental Amalgam Fillings. Amer J Physiol. 258:R939-R945. April 1990.
- Yoshida, M; Satoh, H; Aoyama, H; Kojima, S; Yamamura, Y. Distribution of Mercury in Neonatal Guinea Pigs after Exposure to Mercury Vapor. Bull Environ Contam Toxicol. 43(5):697-704. Nov 1989.

CHAPTER 5

MERCURY DAMAGE TO THE H AND BLOOD VESSELS

Historically, it is well known that exposure to mercury is harmful to the health of humans. Human poisoning from mercury has been documented for over 2300 years, dating back to illness in mercury miners in Roman Spain. Through the centuries, the primary effects of mercury were noted to be neurological, psychological, and oral (gum infection, bone loss and loss of teeth). This unique combination of symptoms is visibly detectable in victims and does not require sophisticated medical testing.

Medical knowledge about cardiovascular disease was minimal prior to the 20th century. In addition, the analysis of cardiovascular disease is dependent upon sophisticated testing based on equally sophisticated research, neither of which was available until the present century. Because of these factors, it isn't surprising that the cardiovascular effects of exposure to mercury were not recognized until fairly recently.

In the mid-19th century Kussmaul had studied the effects of occupational exposure to mercury in workers in mirror factories and the use of mercury in the treatment of syphilis. In 1861 he reported: "Also the activity of the involuntary muscles will be affected. Together with a weakness of the voluntary muscles there will generally be an impairment of the heart. Many observers have noticed that the pulse will be slower. The most common change is great lability; resting rate is 60-70 beats/minute, but at the slightest agitation the rate will rapidly rise to 80-100. Sometimes pronounced tachycardia occurs."

By the 1930's it was recognized that mercury caused damage to the heart and blood vessels. In 1930 Rieselman stated: "One of the most important and most feared consequences of acute mercury poisoning is, as is well known, a paralyzing influence on heart and circulation, followed by reduced blood pressure and death." Rieselman examined workers exposed to mercury and found damage to the heart muscle and changes in nerve regulation of the heart. In 1938 Fellinger and Schweitzer also reported serious vascular damage from mercury exposure and stated that it should be included with the other effects of mercury poisoning.

ealth and Heart Disease

By 1958, reference books, such as von Oettingen's *Poisoning: A Guide to Clinical Diagnosis and Treatment*, stated that cardiac and vascular disturbances were to be found in victims of mercury poisoning. A very interesting report on the use of mercury as a diuretic appeared in 1960. Kahler noted that cardiotoxic effects of mercury diuretics were well known and discussed the attempts to find a mercury compound which had diuretic effects without killing the patient from heart damage. Kahler found that, besides its numerous other effects on the body, mercury caused cardiac arrest (heart attack), preceded by EKG disturbances.

Among the earliest widespread indications of the cardiovascular effects of mercury were in victims of Acrodynia, a disease syndrome known to be caused by mercury. Acrodynia was diagnosed primarily in children who were being exposed to various mercury compounds, mostly a mercurous chloride compound called Calomel, which was commonly used as a teething powder and to combat "diaper rash." Mosby's Medical Dictionary states: "Symptoms include edema, pruritus, generalized skin rash, with pink coloration of the extremities and scarlet coloration of the cheeks and nose, profuse sweating, digestive disturbances, photophobia, polyneuritis, extreme irritability alternating with periods of listlessness and apathy, and failure to thrive. The cause in unknown, although the condition is usually associated with ingestion of or contact with mercury and often with inflammatory changes of obscure origin in the central nervous system."

MERCURY AND HYPERTENSION

In 1952 Vulliamy studied 11 acrodynia victims. Ten of the 11 victims had high blood pressure caused by excessive constriction (narrowing) of arteries. In several experiments on animals, Cheek and associates found that Calomel (mercurous chloride) enhanced the influence of epinephrine (adrenalin) in constricting arteries and causing high blood pressure. In 1953, Warkany and Hubbard found that the therapeutic use of mercury (Calomel) caused hypertension and tachycardia (rapid heartbeat) in children.

Following these observations of cardiovascular events occurring in known human victims of mercury poisoning, medical science researchers began investigations utilizing controlled animal studies.

Beginning in the early 1960's, a group of researchers (led by H.M. Perry, Jr.) at the Washington University School of Medicine in St. Louis began investigating the mechanism by which mercury caused hypertension (high blood pressure). In

Oral Health and Heart Disease

a series of published studies, this group demonstrated that mercury caused the smooth muscles in the walls of arteries to contract, thereby causing hypertension. Various forms of mercury and other metals were introduced into a number of different animals by different means and also applied to isolated strips of aorta. Inorganic mercury caused blood vessel constriction and subsequent hypertension within minutes after exposure. Organic mercury (methylmercury, ethyl mercury) did not! Neither did lead, even in very large quantities. None of the other metals tested (silver, copper, barium, vanadium) were nearly as effective as inorganic mercury in causing hypertension. It was found that the degree of vasoconstriction caused by inorganic mercury was not related to the amount of mercury found in the blood (that is, not dependent on the dose of mercury) and that the degree of hypertension elicited was far greater when the mercury was introduced into arteries or veins than if it was introduced through the gut.

The research of the Washington University group was confirmed by other investigators, including Tomera and Harakal at Temple University School of Medicine and Solomon and Hollenberg at Harvard Medical School. Tomera and Harakal confirmed that organic mercury (methylmercury and ethyl mercury) did not cause the vasoconstriction and high blood pressure found to be caused by inorganic mercury.

Further evidence of the effects of inorganic mercury on the heart and cardiovascular system was produced at Oral Roberts University in Oklahoma and the University of California at Irvine (Rhee and Choi). These researchers found that larger, acute doses of inorganic mercury were so toxic to the heart muscle that severe systemic pathology (low blood pressure) occurred. They also found that inorganic mercury caused actual pathological damage to the heart muscle tissue, which in turn severely decreased heart function to a point that resulted in a dramatic drop in blood pressure.

The phenomenon that smaller amounts of inorganic mercury cause high blood pressure and larger amounts cause cardiac tissue damage with low blood pressure had previously been found by I.M. Trakhtenberg in the Soviet Union.

MERCURY IN SMALL AMOUNTS CAUSES HIGH BLOOD PRESSURE! IN LARGE DOSES IT CAUSES A DANGEROUS DROP IN BLOOD PRESSURE!

d Heart Disease

ND IMPAIRED CARDIAC ELECTRICAL FUNCTION

documentation of the effects of mercury on the cardiovascular sy~~ ans was a study by Dahhan and Orfaly published in the American Journal of Cardiology in 1964. These investigators conducted electrocardiogram tests on 42 victims of organic mercury poisoning in a 1960 Iraq episode. Farmers in Iraq had been issued grain treated with organic mercury fungicides. The grain was intended for planting, but many of the farmers used it for food instead. A serious outbreak of mercury poisoning, including many deaths, resulted from this misuse.

All 42 victims demonstrated ECG changes, denoting damage to the heart. Six had very severe changes, 21 were severe, 10 were moderate, and 5 were slight. Cardiac arrhythmia, abnormal beats of the ventricles, and paroxysmal ventricular tachycardia were also found. These changes were attributed to mercury damage to the heart's pacemaker (the sinoatrial node), the electrical conduction system of the heart, and to reduced blood supply to the heart muscle (myocardial ischemia). (To eliminate any possible confusion regarding the heart effects of organic mercury, it does not cause hypertension, but it does cause major electrical disturbances to normal heart function.)

MERCURY INTERFERES WITH THE ELECTRICAL CONDUCTION PATTERN OF THE HEART!

MERCURY CAUSES HEART DAMAGE

Shortly thereafter, once again, medical scientific researchers performed controlled studies clearly demonstrating that mercury exposure causes interruptions in the electrical conduction pattern of heart function. This research also revealed the actual pathological damage to heart tissue caused by mercury.

In 1968, Kleinfeld and Stein (Maimonides Medical Center in New York and State University of New York) studied the effects of inorganic mercury on animal heart tissue, specifically that in the atrium. Exposing the heart tissue to various concentrations of mercury, as well as other metals, they found that mercury at lower concentrations increased the contraction of the heart muscle by displacing calcium from its normal tissue sites. The displaced calcium then elicited increased heart muscle contraction. At higher concentrations the mercury inhibited the contraction mechanism, thereby reducing heart muscle function. As time went

Oral Health and Heart Disease

by, there was only a partial return to normal function in the m͏͏͏͏ tissues.

In 1977, John Brake and associates at North Carolina State Univer͏ ͏͏͏posed juvenile chickens to various doses of inorganic mercury in the drinking water. Electrocardiographic analyses revealed consistent changes in the electrical conduction patterns of the heart. They also found pathological changes in the heart tissue, including inflammation and fatty degeneration. The authors concluded that low levels of inorganic mercury when administered for even a short period of time can cause pathological changes in the cardiovascular system.

Also in 1977 two Japanese researchers, H.Shiraki and K. Nagashima at Tokyo University Medical School in Japan, investigated the pathology found in human victims of Minimata Disease (which is caused by prolonged exposure to high levels of methylmercury) and also conducted experiments on different animals using radioactive organic and inorganic mercury compounds. The authors observed that the pathology found in mercury poisoning was a result of damage to the blood vessels and subsequent blood supply. Nerve damage resulted from reduced blood flow. They found a thickening of arteries in the victims and hardening of the blood vessels in the brain and other arteries in the body, as well as thrombus (clot) formations in the blood vessels. The victims also demonstrated high blood pressure, damage to heart muscle, and heart attacks. Interestingly, they also showed damage to the Islets of Langerhans in the pancreas, the cells that produce insulin for control of the blood sugar. In this regard, it should be noted that in 1967, T. Wakatsuki had found that in rabbits intoxicated with mercury, there was a conspicuous elevation of blood sugar and blood cholesterol.

In 1990, medical researchers in China investigated the effects of inorganic mercury on the muscles in the wall of the aorta, the major artery leading out of the heart. They found that mercury had a harmful effect that could be related to the development of hardened arteries and high blood pressure.

MERCURY DAMAGES BLOOD VESSELS, INCLUDING THOSE OF THE HEART!

Although ethylmercury and methylmercury are organic mercury compounds, it must be remembered that damage by mercury occurs when it attaches to or enters the cells of the body, no matter what form the mercury is in when it enters the body. Ethylmercury and methylmercury are very toxic forms of mercury because they easily enter the body and its cells. Mercury vapor is also very toxic for the same reason.

In 1974, a very interesting document appeared in the United States. It was published by the National Institutes of Health branch of the Public Health Service of the U.S. Department of Health, Education, and Welfare. It is entitled *Chronic Effects of Mercury on Organisms* by I.M. Trakhtenberg of the U.S.S.R. The document is a 333 page account of extensive research conducted in the Soviet Union on the effects of chronic exposure to mercury and its compounds. An entire chapter is devoted to the effects of mercury on the cardiovascular system.

Armed with the knowledge that mercury readily binds to the thiol (sulfur/hydrogen combination) site of living tissues, the Soviet researchers investigated mercury's toxic action on a wide range of tissues, including those of the cardiovascular system. They found that mercury affected several aspects of cardiac function, including the ability of heart muscle to contract, the electrical conduction activity in the heart, and the function of regulators of cardiac activity.

The cardiovascular effects of chronic exposure to low levels of mercury vapor were studied in a clinical-statistical study of 656 subjects. The subjects exhibited an increased occurrence of rapid heart beat, irregular pulse, chest pains, heart palpitations, and high blood pressure. The majority of the subjects with cardiovascular problems were over age 40, but a large number of such cases were among the 20-29 age group.

In four other Russian studies of subjects who worked around mercury, Trakhtenberg reported that the percentage of workers with high blood pressure or low blood pressure were 42%, 60%, 44.4%, 50% (males), and 68% (females).

Trakhtenberg conducted an experiment on rabbits exposed to low doses of mercury vapor compared to control animals who were not exposed. He monitored cardiac response by electrocardiogram (ECG). During the first 3-4 weeks of exposure there were no changes. Then rapid heart beat was encountered, followed by diminished heart beat. By the third month of exposure all of the exposed rabbits exhibited slow heart beat and abnormal ECG changes, especially a decrease in the force of the contraction.

Further experiments by Trakhtenberg demonstrated that mercury blocked the ability of the heart to respond to stimulation of the Vagus Nerve (a nerve from the brain responsible for maintaining the heart beat). It was found that mercury blocked the action of acetylcholine, the neurotransmitter that passes the nerve

Oral Health and Heart Disease

impulse from the Vagus Nerve to the heart muscle. Both acetylcholin nerve receptors in the heart muscle contain thiol (sulfur/hydrogen) proteins. When mercury attached to the thiol protein in the heart muscle receptors and in the acetylcholine, the heart muscle could not receive the Vagus Nerve electrical impulse required for contraction.

NEUROTRANSMITTERS!

Besides this peripheral effect on the heart contraction, Trakhtenberg reported that Soviet investigators had also found that mercury caused functional changes in centers regulating cardiac activity and directly to the heart muscle itself. They found that mercury accumulated in the heart muscle and heart valves, causing damage by attaching to thiols of proteins. This damage was indicated by ECG changes and confirmed by histologic study. The damage was found in the coronary arteries and capillaries supplying blood to the heart tissue and in the heart muscle itself.

MERCURY DAMAGES HEART MUSCLE TISSUE, BLOOD VESSELS, AND HEART VALVES!

The Russian investigators also found that mercury affected heart function by influencing the hormones from the pituitary gland (called "pituitrin"). Pituitrin contains several active hormones that have a profound and important influence on the body, including one that affects the constriction of arteries. They administered pituitrin to test animals, with and without accompanying low dose mercury administration and measured the effects by ECG analysis. They found that the test animals developed coronary insufficiency at lower doses of pituitrin than did the control animals. In animals subjected to prolonged exposure to low doses of mercury, the ECG changes were sharply developed and the cardiovascular function was inhibited.

MERCURY AFFECTS HORMONES THAT REGULATE THE HEART!

A number of published scientific studies on animals have confirmed the harmful effects of mercury on the cardiovascular system. In 1980, a study by L. B. Jha and B. Bhatia at the Jawaharal Nehru University, in New Delhi, India found that mercuric chloride caused a reduction in the blood flow to the coronary arteries that supply the heart (vasoconstriction). As stated previously, research had already demonstrated that mercury does cause this constriction of arteries by contracting the muscle tissue in the artery walls. The reduction or blockage of blood supply to the heart muscle is what causes angina and heart attacks (myocardial infarction). The contraction of the arterial muscle tissue was caused by mercury's interference with the required activity of sodium and potassium.

MERCURY CONSTRICTS THE CORONARY ARTERIES THAT SUPPLY BLOOD TO THE HEART TISSUE!

In 1983 and 1984 M. Carmignani and associates at the Catholic University in Rome, Italy and the University of Cincinnati Medical Center, in Cincinnati, Ohio, published the results of their animal research. They monitored aortic blood pressure, heart rate, electrocardiogram, and rate or pressure in the left ventricle of the heart in control animals and test animals exposed to chronic low doses of inorganic mercury (mercuric chloride). These investigators found that chronic exposure to mercury affected cardiovascular function by interfering with the body mechanisms that regulated blood pressure and cardiovascular regulating hormones (dopamine, epinephrine, and). [Note: Epinephrine and norepinephrine are also called"adrenalin" and "noradrenalin."] They determined that mercury exposure increased the force of heart muscle contraction, causing high blood pressure in the test animals. These actions of mercury were explained by its blocking the passage of calcium ions into the heart muscle cells. Their research continued and in 1989 they concluded that the alterations in cardiovascular function caused by mercury were from combined effects on the nerves, hormones, cell metabolism, and possibly even the immune system.

Further evidence of the harmful effects of mercury on the cardiovascular system were determined from laboratory experiments by Wierzbicki and associates at the Medical School of Lodz, in Lodz, Poland in 1983. They found that low concentrations of various mercury compounds accelerated the blood coagulation. They stated, "Due to industrial and environmental pollution with mercury and a common appearance of blood circulation diseases, pathological changes in blood coagulation accompanying mercury intoxication seem to be an unquestionably important problem to investigate." These astute researchers have opened the door to an area of needed research that could have a monumental impact on the health of mankind!

Oral Health and Heart Disease

This effect of mercury on blood clotting was confirmed by research conducted by Kostka and associates in 1989.

MERCURY CAUSES BLOOD TO CLOT FASTER AND EASIER!

Very little formal research can be found that investigated the actual pathological affects of pre-natal mercury exposure on the cardiovascular system. One interesting study was published by T.F. Gale in 1980. He injected pregnant hamsters with one single dose of inorganic mercury on day seven, eight, or nine of gestation and compared the results to control animals not receiving mercury. The pre-natal mercury exposure produced marked toxicity to the babies, including a high incidence of abnormal hearts, characterized by dilation of the heart with a thinning and weakening of the heart walls. It has been scientifically proven that inhaled mercury vapor penetrates the placental membrane far more thoroughly than does inorganic mercury, thereby greatly increasing the potential for this fetal damage. Further, Dr. M.J. Vimy and his colleagues at the University of Calgary Medical School in Canada have scientifically proven that unborn babies are highly exposed to mercury from their mothers' dental amalgam fillings.

In 1980 Orlowski and Mercer published the results of their investigation of six victims of Mucocutaneous Lymph Node Syndrome (Kawasaki Disease). They pointed out that the occurrence of MLNS in the United States paralleled the increasing concern with environmental pollution of natural bodies of water with mercury. They also emphasized the similarities of the disease to Acrodynia, a disease known to be caused by mercury, and felt that MLNS might represent a disease related to environmental poisoning from mercury. They compared the urine mercury levels of the six patients to matched control subjects and found the levels to be abnormally high in the six MLNS victims. They also found that the MLNS victims had high aneurysm occurrences of the coronary arteries of the heart, electrocardiogram alterations and even myocardial infarctions due to blockage of the coronary arteries.

DENTAL AMALGAM AND CARDIOVASCULAR DISEASE

The new awareness of chronic mercury exposure from dental amalgam fillings has already stimulated the medical scientific community to begin investigations of potential harmful effects, including those to the cardiovascular system.

Oral Health and Heart Disease

A recently published study by Siblerud investigated the cardiovascular status of subjects with and without mercury amalgam fillings. Subjects with amalgam fillings had significantly higher blood pressure, lower heart rate, lower hemoglobin levels, and lower percentages of red blood cells. They also had a greater incidence of chest pains, rapid heart beat (tachycardia), anemia, fatigue, tiring easily, and being tired in the morning. The author stated that the study suggested that inorganic mercury poisoning from dental amalgam does affect the cardiovascular system. This initial study will hopefully stimulate other medical scientists to investigate the issue.

SUMMARY

For more than 75 years scientific evidence demonstrating the widespread cardiovascular effects of inorganic mercury and mercury vapor has been accumulating. These effects can result in arrhythmia, hypertension, impaired cardiac electrical and neurotransmitter function, pathological changes in heart muscle tissue, damage to blood vessels and heart valves, constriction of coronary arteries and increased potential for blood clots.

During this same period of time scientific evidence has also accumulated showing that silver/mercury dental fillings release mercury vapor and abraded particles of mercury over the life of the fillings. It has now been firmly established that individuals with silver/mercury amalgam dental fillings experience significant mercury exposure to the tissues of the cardiovascular system. In spite of all of the published scientific evidence of the damage caused by mercury to the cardiovascular system, as yet there has been only one controlled study investigating a possible connection of chronic mercury exposure to the occurrence of cardiovascular disease in human population groups. We fervently hope that the revelation of this evidence will stimulate additional research and perhaps discover that mercury may in fact be the "missing link" in the devastating occurrence of heart disease.

Oral Health and Heart Disease

REFERENCES:

- Brake, J; Thaxton, P; Hestor, PY. Mercury Induced Cardiovascular Abnormalities in the Chicken. Arch Environ Contam Toxicol. 6:269-77. 1977.

- Carmignani, M. et al. Mechanisms in Cardiovascular Regulation Following Exposure of Male Rats to Inorganic Mercury. Toxicol. Appl. Pharmacol. 69:442-50. 1983.

- Carmignani, M. & Boscolo, P. Cardiovascular Homeostasis in Rats Chronically Exposed to Mercuric Chloride. Arch. Toxicol. Suppl. 7. 383-8. 1984.

- Carmignani, M. et al. Renal Ultrastructural Alterations and Cardiovascular Changes in Rats Exposed to Mercuric Chloride. Arch Toxicol. Suppl 13:353-6. 1989.

- Cheek, DB & Wu, F. Effect of Calomel on Plasma Epinephrine in Rat and Relationship to Mechanisms in Pink Disease. Arch Dis Childhood. 34:502-4. 1959.

- Cheek, DB et al. Effect of Mercurous Chloride (Calomel) and Epinephrine (Sympathetic Stimulation) on Rats: Importance of Findings to Mechanisms in Infantile Acrodynia (Pink Disease). Pediatrics. 23:302-13. 1959.

- Dahhan, SS. & Orfaly, H. Electrocardiographic Changes in Mercury Poisoning. American J. Cardiology. 14:178-83. August 1964.

- Fellinger, K; Schweitzer, F. Gefasserkrankungen nach Quecksilbervergiftungen. Arch Gewerbepath Gewerbehyg. 9:269-75. 1938.

- Gale, TF. Cardiac and Non-cardiac Malformations Produced by Mercury in Hamsters. Bull. Environ. Contam. Toxicol. 25:726-32. 1980.

- Jha, LB. & Bhatia, B. Effect of Mercuric Chloride on Coronary Flow in Perfused Rat Heart. Bull. Environ. Contam. Toxicol. 31(2): 132-8. 1883.

- Kahler, HJ. Zur Frage der Kardiotoxischen Wirkung des Quecksilbers, inbesondere des Saatfruchtbeizmittel "Ceresan". Zbl Arbeitsmed Arbeitsschutz. 10:25-31. 1960.

- Kleinfeld, M; Stein, E. Action of Divalent Cations on Membrane Potentials and Contractility in Rat Atrium. Amer J Physiol. 215(3):593-9. Sept 1968.

- Kostka, B; Michalski, M; Krajewska, U; Wierzbicki, R. Blood Coagulation Changes in Rats Poisoned with Methylmercuric Chloride (MeHg). Pol J Pharmacol Pharm. 41(2):183-9. Mar-Apr 1989.

- Kussmaul, A. Untersuchungen ueber den constitutionellen Mercurialismus und sein Verhaeltniss zur constitutionellen Syphilis. Wuerzburg. 1861.

- Lu, KP; Zhao, SH; Wang, DS. The Stimulatory Effect of Heavy Metal Cations on Proliferation of Aortic Smooth Muscle Cells. Sci China [B]. 33(3):303-10. Mar 1990.

- Maurissen, JPJ. History of Mercury and Mercurialism. New York State J. Medicine. pp. 1902-09. December 1981.

- Mosby's Revised 2nd Edition, Medical Dictionary. The C.V. Mosby Co. St. Louis, MO, 1987.

- Oettingen, WFvon. Poisoning: A Guide to Clinical Diagnosis and Treatment. 2nd Ed. Saunders Co. London. 1958.

Oral Health and Heart Disease

- Orlowski, JP & Mercer, RD. Urine Mercury Levels in Kawasaki Disease. Pediatrics. 66(4): 633-6. October 1980.
- Perry, HM, Jr.; Yunice, A. Acute Pressor Effects of Intra-Arterial Cadmium and Mercuric Ions in Anesthetized Rats. Proc Soc Exp Biol Med. 120:805-8. 1965.
- Perry, HM, Jr.; Schoepfle, E; Bourgoignie, J. In Vitro Production and Inhibition of Aortic Vasoconstriction by Mercuric, Cadmium, and Other Metal Ions. Proc Soc Exp Biol Med. 124:485-90. 1967.
- Perry, HM, Jr.; Erlanger, M; Yunice, A; Schoepfle, E. Perry, EF. Hypertension and Tissue Metal Levels Following Intravenous Cadmium, Mercury, and Zinc. Amer J Physiol. 219:755-61. Sep 1970.
- Perry, HM, Jr.; Erlanger, M. Hypertension and Tissue Metal Levels After Intraperitoneal Cadmium, Mercury, and Zinc. Amer J Physiol. 220:808-11. March 1971.
- Rhee, HM; Choi, BH. Hemodynamic and Electrophysiological Effects of Mercury in Intact Anesthetized Rabbits and in Isolated perfused Hearts. Exp Molec Pathol. 50:281-90. 1989.
- Rieselman, SD. Einfluss der Quecksilberintoxikation auf die inneren Organe. Arch Gewerbepathol. 1:496. 1930.
- Shiraki, H & Nagashima, K. Essential Neuropathology of Alkylmercury Intoxications in Humans from the Acute to the Chronic Stage With Special Reference to Experimental Whole Body Autoradiographic Study Using Labeled Mercury Compounds. Neurotox. Ed: Roizin, L, et al. 247-60. 1977.
- Siblerud, RL. The Relationship Between Mercury from Dental Amalgam and the Cardiovascular System. Sci Tot Environ. 99:23-35. 1990.
- Solomon, HS; Hollenberg, NK. Catecholamine Release: Mechanism of Mercury-Induced Vascular Smooth Muscle Contraction. Amer J Physiol. 229(1):8-12. July 1975.
- Tomera, JF; Harakal, C. Mercury- and Lead-Induced Contraction of Aortic Smooth Muscle In Vitro. Arch Int Pharmacodyn. 283(2):295-302. Oct 1986.
- Trakhtenberg, IM. Chronic Effects of Mercury on Organisms. Chap. VI:109-34. The Micromercurialism Phenomenon in Mercury Handlers. Chap. XI:199-210. Cardiotoxic Effects of Mercury. DHEW Publ. No, (NIH) 74-473. 1974.
- Vimy, MJ: Takahashi, Y: Lorscheider, FL. Maternal-fetal Distribution of Mercury (203Hg) Released From Dental Amalgam Fillings. Amer J Physiol. 258:R939-R945. April 1990.
- Vulliamy, GD. Vasomotor Disturbance in Pink Disease. Lancet. 2:1248-51. 1952.
- Wakatsuki, T. Inapparent intoxication with special reference to pesticides of organic mercurial origin. Psychiatr. Neurol Jpn., 69:1004-1106, 1967.
- Warkany, J; Hubbard, DM. Acrodynia and Mercury. J Pediatrics. 42:365-386. 1953
- Wierzbicki R., Et al. Interaction of fibrinogen With Mercury. Thrombo Res 30(6):579-585. 1983.

CHAPTER 6
THINGS YOU CAN DO

Periodontitis

Let's operate on the premise that YOU are at least partly to blame for having a periodontal problem. So how do you start to begin reversing the conditions that created the problem in the first place? As you know we are dealing with bacteria as a causal factor, and our immediate concern should be taking actions that will decrease the oral bacteria count. Actions you can take personally involve: tooth brushing; tooth paste selection; use of an antiseptic mouthwash; use of an oral irrigator; topical applications of antibacterial products; restricting or reducing use of substances that may be injurious to the oral tissues; establishing a plan to have necessary dental work done, when it is financially feasible. Lets examine these items in more detail:

Brushing your teeth

This simple act involves a tremendous amount of advertising hype that we are all subjected to. Thankfully, the tooth brush itself has developed into a viable instrument employing the latest technology in materials and design. Consequently, you just need to pick one that has medium or soft bristles without too much regard for brand name. In this day and age, you should seriously consider using a power tooth brush as the prices have reached a level that makes them affordable to most individuals. Three primary considerations in brushing your teeth should be reduction or prevention of additional plaque or tartar forming, reduction of oral bacteria and massaging of the gum tissue.

Sonic and power toothbrushes are proliferating and there have been several studies comparing different brands and types. In one study involving two different sonic toothbrushes the authors concluded that compared to a manual toothbrush the sonic brushes were more effective in removing plaque and preventing gingivitis.(1) There was also an investigation of whether power toothbrushes could remove plaque and also reduce pain in dentin hypersensitivity. There was a 35-40% reduction in pain as compared to the baseline data. A round rotary brush and a straight sonic brush were used in the study and there was not

Oral Health and Heart Disease

a significant statistical difference in the results of both brushes.(2) Conversely, there are studies showing rotary brushes more effective than sonic brushes and vice versa.(3-4) We think the bottom line is, regardless of the type, power brushes are a real adjunct to reducing plaque, inflammation and stimulating your gum tissue..

Reduction of plaque

This aspect is accomplished primarily by the physical act of brushing itself, without consideration of the type or brand of toothpaste used. In other words, you are mechanically trying to get rid of any buildup that hasn't hardened into calculus yet, and toothpaste is not a requisite to accomplish this. In this regard, the information provided in the previous paragraph about power tooth brushes greatly simplifies your task of helping to keep plaque under control.

In his current Newsletter "Alternatives for the health - conscious individual" Dr. David G. Williams used an article he had obtained from the Price-Pottenger Foundation (1-800-366-3748) as the basis for a portion of his newsletter dealing with periodontal disease and the heart. (Vol. 8, No. 24, June 2001. You can buy this issue by calling 1-800-219-8591. Or if you would like to subscribe to this outstanding monthly health newsletter the price is $69.00 per year)

The article was by Dr. John E. Waters, DDS and was titled "Correctable Systematic Disorders Indicated by Presence of Salivary Calculus."(5) Dr. Waters graduated from dental school in 1918 and for the first ten years of dental practice, accepted what he had been taught that calculus caused pyorrhea (periodontitis) and it should be removed as required to prevent pyorrhea from occurring.

After ten years of private practice Dr. Waters established a Dental Staff in a County Hospital. This gave him the opportunity to study patients in groups according to their medical problems. As a direct result of his observations he determined that diabetic and cancer patients, and most of the patients on the chronic disease wards, all had very heavy build-ups of calculus and inflammation of the gum tissue.

He began to investigate and try to determine what caused these groups of patients to have so much calculus and gum disease. In this context, in January 1931, Dr. Waters enrolled in a long course of post-graduate study in dental nutrition under Harold F. Hawkins DDS, at the College of Dentistry, University of Southern California. He discussed his observations about calculus with Dr. Hawkins who

Oral Health and Heart Disease

became very interested. Dr. Hawkins told him about a particular case in his own practice that fitted into Dr. Water's observations: A lady who had been diagnosed with cancer of the cervix and uterus and who had received a single radium treatment. A short time later she saw her dentist who noted excessive calculus and referred her for a nutritional consultation with Dr. Hawkins. Evidently the program Dr. Hawkins put her on was very effective because to the best of his knowledge she became calculus-free and remained so thereafter. Approximately a year later the lady went back to the Cancer Clinic for a check-up and further treatment if required. No evidence of cancer could be found, nor of the former presence of one. Other members of the Clinic were called in to see the cancer case "that a single radium treatment had cured."

In discussing his own wife's calculus forming problems and her fears of getting cancer, Dr. Hawkins suggested a defective fat metabolism as being the etiological factor involved, probably a liver deficiency. Therefore, starting in 1931 his wife was given 10 grains of ox-bile after each meal. The result was an almost total absence of calculus formation.

After World War II, Dr. Waters began evaluating every patient that entered his practice as well as referring those with calculus to his personal physician for further medical evaluation. Dr. Waters found that 90 percent of his patients who had calculus problems did not like the taste of fatty meats. After consultation with physicians and nutritionists he concluded that people who do not like fat are not able to assimilate fats and consequently, develop a dislike for them, without ever knowing the underlying reason.

From Dr. Hawkins he gathered the following impressions of what occurs in this syndrome.:

"There appears to be in certain fats a factor, let us call it factor F for simplicity, which controls the selective function of the kidneys in selecting from the blood stream the acid wastes of life's processes, and eliminating them via the urine. When factor F is not adequate in the diet the acid waste is not eliminated properly. It remains in the blood stream to result in systemic acidosis; the saliva in turn being made from that more than normally acid blood, precipitates solids on the teeth in the form known as dental calculus."

"This factor F does not appear to be in vegetable fats, pork fats, or some others. It is present in beef, mutton and poultry fats, and probably in whale, seal, walrus

Oral Health and Heart Disease

and other animal fats on the Arctic, as Eskimos and others using such fats have been reported as being quite free from dental calculus."

When the patient's physician found nothing wrong, Dr. Waters would prescribe ox-bile to be taken after each meal to correct what was an apparent inadequate supply of bile from the liver to handle fats. He suggested two 5 grain tablets to be taken after each meal. If the patient got diarrhea from two tablets, the dose was to be reduced to one tablet after each meal. If diarrhea persists, treatment should be discontinued, the diarrhea indicating an excess of bile and disproving a bile deficiency. If use of the ox-bile does not result in diarrhea then the diagnosis of a bile deficiency has been confirmed, and the procedure has been a safe simple and inexpensive diagnostic measure. When diarrhea results, some other cause for the impaired fat metabolism must be sought.

Subsequent to 1932, Dr. Waters, has not found a single confirmed cancer patient he came in contact with who did not also have the dental calculus problem. Although his observation of cancer patients is limited the relationship demands further exploration.

Why this tremendously important research has been ignored and not expanded upon and replicated is certainly a mystery. Here it appears is the key to stopping periodontal problems before they even start by decreasing or eliminating plaque. The definition of dental plaque is: "a soft thin film of food debris, mucin and dead epithelial cells deposited on the teeth, providing the medium for the growth of various bacteria. The main inorganic components are calcium and phosphorus with small amounts of magnesium, potassium, and sodium; the organic matrix consists of polysaccharides, proteins, carbohydrates, lipids, and other components. Plaque plays an important etiologic role in the development of dental caries and periodontal and gingival diseases and provides the base for the development of materia alba; calcified plaque forms dental calculus. (Materia alba is a whitish or cream-colored cheesy mass deposited around the necks of the teeth, composed of food debris, mucin and dead epithelial cells)" definitions taken from Dorland's Medical Dictionary.

Your local health food store should have some bile salt products. Dr. Williams, in his newsletter, recommended using a product from Standard Process called *Cholacol*. However, it is only available through health care professionals. You can ask your dentist, physician, or chiropractor to order them for you. Or, you can call Standard Process at 800-558-8740 for a doctor referral near you.

Oral Health and Heart Disease

Toothpaste

This is a delicate issue to bring up because of the fluoride controversy. If fluoride incorporation into toothpaste was your only exposure to this very toxic substance it might be acceptable. However, you are inundated with fluoride, especially if you live in a community with fluoridated water. Unfortunately, after 50 plus years of water fluoridation epidemiology studies have shown that children living in areas without water fluoridation have fewer or the same number of cavities without having to continually swallow a poison added to their water.(6) More importantly, the Centers for Disease Control (CDC) has recently acknowledged that fluoride's mechanism of action is primarily topical and not systemic.(7) This means you don't need to swallow fluoride to reap its **TINY** benefits.

Furthermore, most people are not aware that over 90% of the fluoride added to water is an industrial waste product generated from the phosphate fertilizer industry that contains a number of impurities including arsenic, lead, chromium, cadmium and barium.(8) Most major brand name toothpastes all include fluoride, supposedly as an antibacterial agent. However, a recent UNICEF report questions the validity of that premise "...Fluoride inhibits enzymes that breed acid-producing oral bacteria whose acid eats away tooth enamel. This observation is valid, but some scientists now believe that the harmful impact of fluoride on other useful enzymes far outweighs the beneficial effect on caries prevention."(9) Enough said about fluoride. If you are interested in getting more information about the fluoride issue we recommend that you visit Dr. Paul Connett's web site http:www.fluoridealert.org. **(Be sure you use the "org" category, because the American Dental Association (ADA) has acquired the name and URL for www.fluoridealert.com.** If you use the "com" category, you will get the ADA site telling you all about the wonderful things fluoride does for you, rather than the truth about this toxic material).

As we see it, the greatest benefit that could be achieved from a toothpaste would be if it contained ingredients that would kill bacteria and viruses and yet be tissue friendly, not damaging any of the oral mucosa. Excluding those that contain fluoride greatly narrows the selection. In recent years there have been several toothpastes introduced that have incorporated many beneficial herbs and essential oils. To name a few: *Neem Tooth Paste*, a herbal/ayurvedic tooth paste; *Desert Essence Tea Tree Oil Toothpaste - Ginger*; *Auromere's Ayurvedic Formula*; *Herbal Toothpaste and Gum Therapy®* by The Natural Dentist® *Tooth and Gum Paste* from Dental Herb Co.,Inc. The first four should be available at your local health food store; however, *Tooth and Gum Paste* can only be ordered from a dentist or physician who have it available in their office. (you can call 1-800-747-4372 for a doctor near you who stocks the product).

Antiseptics and antimicrobials

As there is no television or newspaper hype and marketing program, few people outside of those that work in hospitals or medical offices, are aware of a product called Betadine. Betadine, is a 1% Povidone Iodine (a complex produced by reacting iodine with the polymer povidone, which slowly releases iodine) that is water solubilized which is why it does not sting the healthy or inflamed/infected oral mucosa. It does not discolor the teeth and tongue or effect your taste sensation. The only contraindication is possible iodine allergy. Prior to 1991, although used extensively in gynecology and dermatology, it had not been used for periodontitis. However, since then there have been many studies published in peer reviewed medical and dental journals demonstrating its efficacy in eliminating oral bacteria and viruses and reducing or preventing bacteremia associated with various dental procedures.(10-12)

Antiseptics that are locally applied gain in significance due to their reliable microbicidal effectiveness and the fact that there is a rising incidence of highly resistant bacteria. Oral intake of antibiotics to treat a problem systemically are not sufficient to eradicate superficial surface bacteria and locally applied antibiotics can cause new resistance rapidly. Following is a list of products that have either or all of these characteristics: antibacterial, anti-inflammatory, antiviral and tissue regeneration.

Tooth and Gum Tonic (mouthwash) and *Under The Gum Irrigant* (for use with irrigation devices) by Dental Herb Co. Both of these products are alcohol free and are made without chemicals. They contain herbs and essential oils that have been used for centuries to maintain healthy tissues which for the first time have been combined into a unique and proprietary formula to maintain good oral hygiene. As stated previously for the toothpaste, these products can only be purchased through a dentist who stocks them. Call 1-800-747-4372 to locate a dental office near you that carries the products. A word of caution, none of these products should be used by children under 12 years of age.

Herbal Mouth and Gum Therapy® mouthrinse by The Natural Dentist.® This mouthwash in scientific studies has been shown clinically effective in reducing

Oral Health and Heart Disease

gingivitis and plaque. This product is available at most health food stores and some drug store chains.(13)

Grapefruit Seed Extract by NurtiBiotics®. The product contains CITRICIDAL®. CITRICIDAL is synthesized from organically grown grapefruit. The process converts the grapefruit bioflavonoids into an extremely potent compound that has proven highly effective in addressing oral hygiene problems. It comes in a liquid concentrate and also in capsule form. You cannot apply the liquid directly to the skin but you can make a solution using 3-15 drops that is very effective as a mouthwash.

FoliCare™ Oral Care Rinse by AMNI® (Advanced Medical Nutrition, Inc.). This product is based on several research studies demonstrating a local beneficial effect on gingivitis rather than a systemic effect. A 1% solution of folate was utilized and study subjects rinsed for one minute before spitting it out.(14-15)

Propolis Extract. Propolis has been used since ancient times in folk medicine for its beneficial effects. It is a mixture of resin, essential oils and waxes mixed with bee glue; also it contains amino acid, minerals, ethanol, vitamin A, B Complex, E, Pollen and a highly active ingredient known as Bioflavonoid.(16) There is a substantive database on the biological activity and toxicity of propolis indicating it may have many antibiotic, antifungal, antiviral and antitumor properties. Although reports of allergic reaction are not uncommon, propolis is relatively non-toxic.(17) However, for someone who has never used Propolis before, it might be wise to do a simple evaluation by placing some on your skin and see if you have any reaction.

MistORAL™ is an oral spray for gingivitis. It was formulated by Dr. Jonathan Wright and Dr. Donald Carter as a topical mouth spray and it has produced significant results in those suffering from periodontal disease. This is the first time all of these nutrients have been put together in one product. The efficacy of active ingredients in this oral spray have been substantiated in peer-reviewed scientific studies. In addition to using it after brushing, the neat thing about this product is that you can carry it with you to use during the day when you are unable to brush. MistOral is available from the Life Extension Foundation by calling 1-800-544-4440 or you can order online at http://www.lef.org.

Oral Health and Heart Disease

Oral Irrigation Devices

These are powered devices with a pump and a well or enclosure where liquid can be placed that can subsequently be pumped through flexible plastic tubing to a hand piece that allows you to direct the flow of liquid to any location in the mouth. Tooth brushing and rinsing alone do not reach pathogens residing in periodontal pockets of increased depths, oral hygiene procedures should include subgingival treatment with a home oral irrigator.

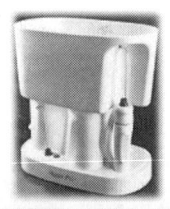

Waterpik is carried by most drug store chains and super markets and can also be purchased directly on-line from Waterpik. Their web site offers a greater variety of models than are normally available at retail outlets. http://www.waterpik.com/products/

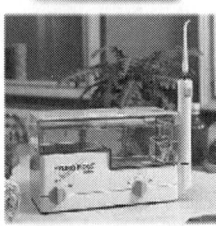

Hydro Floss is primarily sold through dental offices or can be purchased on-line from Hydro Floss. The major difference between the two units is that Hydro Floss incorporates a patented principle of magneto-hydro-dynamics which gives a 44% greater reduction in plaque than with non-magnetic oral irrigators. However, there is a substantial price difference. http://www.hydrofloss.com/

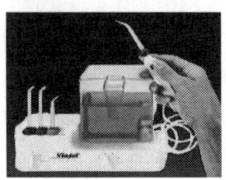

Via-Jet 7500 Oral Irrigator May be purchased through dental offices, or on-line at http://www.viajet.com. This is the *OraTec* site which is the company that provides the phase contrast microscope systems to dentists. They also feature an array of homecare products, including battery operated portable irrigators that are great for trips or work

Whether you are actively treating existing periodontal disease or, whether you are simply doing preventive oral hygiene to preclude getting periodontal disease, adding an oral irrigator to your regimen can make a significant difference in achieving your desired objective. They are very versatile as they give you the ability to put astringents, antibacterial solutions, oral rinses or mouthwash into the irrigator well and put the solution directly into the periodontal pockets, or around the gum line of each tooth. Irrigators have a variable control that permits you to select the amount of pressure or force of the liquid being pushed out of the nozzle and into the pocket.

Oral Health and Heart Disease

We believe it is important to always use some type of antimicrobial solution with your irrigator as there has been some research indicating it is possible to produce a transient bacteremia using plain water, pushing the bacteria in the periodontal pocket into the tissue. Use of antimicrobial solutions eliminates or minimizes this probability. In this same context, it is also very important that you only use a gentle pressure. Excessive pressures have the potential of damaging your gum tissues and possibly causing transient bacteremia. This is especially true if you are treating an active periodontal condition.

There are probably other brand name oral irrigators on the market. However, the three brands that seem to be the most popular are ***Waterpik*** and ***Hydro Floss*** and ***ViaJet***. ViaJet is available from distributors other than OraTec and may be found on the Internet by using the search term "viajet oral irrigator."

REFERENCES:

1. Zimmer S, Fosca M, Roulet JF. Clinical study of the effectiveness of two sonic toothbrushes. J Clin Dent 2000;11(1):24-27.

2. Hefti AF, Stone C. Power toothbrushes, gender, and dentin hypersensitivity. Clin Oral Investig 2000 Jun;4(2):91-97.

3. Sarker S, McLey L, Boyd RL. Clinical and laboratory evaluation of powered electric toothbrushes: laboratory determination of relative interproximal cleaning efficiency of four powered toothbrushes. J Clin Dent 1997;8(3 Spec No):81-85.

4. Ho HP, Niederman R. Effectiveness of the Sonicare sonic toothbrush on reduction of plaque, gingivitis, probing pocket depth and subgingival bacteria in adolescent orthodontic patients. J Cin Dent 1997;8(Spec No):15-19.

5. Waters, John E., DDS. Correctable systematic disorders indicated by presence of salivary calculus. PPNF Health Journal. Vol. 21, No. 2.

6. Brunelle JA, Carlos JP. Recent trends in dental caries in U.S. children and the effect of water fluoridation. J Dent Res 1990 Feb;69:723-727

7. Centers for Disease Control "Achievements in Public Health 1900-1999. Fluoridation of Drinking Water to Prevent Caries," MORBIDITY AND MORTALITY WEEKLY REPORT VOL 48, No 41 (October 22, 1999) pages 933-940.

8. IFIN Bulletin #228: Fluoridation & Arsenic. International Fluoride Infromation Network http://www.fluoridealert.org

9. UNICEF Water Environment & Sanitation (WES) http://www.unicef.org/programme/wes/info/fluor.htm

10. Kovesi G. The use of Betadine antiseptic in the treatment of oral surgical, parodontological and oral mucosal diseases. Fogorv SZ 1999 Aug;92:243-250

11. Wichelhaus TA., et al. Antibacterial effectiveness of povidone-iodine (Betaisodona) against highly resistance gram positive organisms. Zentralbl Hyg Umweltmed 1998 Feb;200(5-6):435-442. (article in German)

12. Kawana R. et al. Inactivation of human viruses by povidone-iodine in comparison with other antiseptics. Dermatology 1997;195 Suppl 2:29-35.

13. Kaim JM, Gultz J, DoL, Scherer W. An in vitro investigation of the antimicrobial activity of an herbal mouthrinse. J Clin Dent 1998;9(2):46-48.

14. Thomson ME, Pack AR. Effects of extended systemic and topical folate supplementation on gingivitis of pregnancy. J Clin Periodontol 1982 May;9(3):275-280.

15. Pack AR. Folate mouthwash effects on established gingivitis in periodontal patients. J Clin Periodontol 1984 Oct;11(9):619-628.

Oral Health and Heart Disease

16. Mahmoud AS, Almas K, Dahlan AA. The effect of propolis on dentinal hypersensitivity and level of satisfaction among patients from a university hospital Riyadh, Saudi Arabia. Indian J Dent Res 1999 Oct-Dec;10(4):130-137.
17. Burdock GA. Review of the biological properties and toxicity of bee propolis (propolis). Food Chem Toxicol 1998 Apr;36(4):47-63.

Oral Health and Heart Disease

Chapter 7
Nutritional Support For A Healthy Mouth And Heart

In 1969 a study was published that had evaluated the use of multivitamin supplements to determine what effect they might have on tooth mobility and gingival sulcus depth. The study concluded that the multivitamin supplement did in fact reduce the sulcus depth, reduce tooth mobility and improved the gingival state.(1) That study was published over 30 years ago, and little if anything has subsequently been done by the dental establishment to further the use of nutritional supplements to treat periodontal disease or improve periodontal health. Fortunately though, we now have one commercial company that has developed and tested a nutritional formula to fill this void. (See page 72)

The nutrients listed in this chapter are in random sequence and are not in any order of priority of their importance to oral health.

Vitamin C

"Is antiscorbutic, antioxidant, antistress, and a detoxificant of heavy metals and pesticides. Promotes formation of collagen (a protein that forms the basis for connective tissue, the most abundant tissue in the body). Helps maintain the integrity of osteoid tissue of bone, and dentin of teeth. It is essential for wound healing and facilitates recovery from burns. Vitamin C is involved in the absorption and utilization of iron and in the utilization and metobolism of folic acid, phenylalanine and tyrosine. Vitamin C is stored in the adrenal glands and is essential in the formation of adrenalin. It also helps in the maintenance of capillaries."(2)

In a study using young men as the subjects, their vitamin C status was purposely depleted to see the effect on the gingiva. The propensity of the gingiva to become inflamed or bleed on probing was reduced after taking only 65 mg/day during repletion of their vitamin C status.(3)

What these researchers demonstrated by depleting vitamin C levels was the development of classic symptoms of scurvy. The Scottish surgeon James Lind is credited with discovering in 1744 that symptoms of bleeding and rotting gums

Oral Health and Heart Disease

experienced by sailors at sea could be alleviated by oranges and lemons and to some degree, apple cider. It wasn't until 1930 that the substance that actually was curing scurvy was identified as ascorbic acid, commonly referred to as vitamin C.

So, if your gums bleed easily, chances are you have a vitamin C deficiency. As scurvy progresses, there is a loss of periodontal support which leads to tooth loosening. Diminished collagen synthesis resulting from a vitamin C deficiency may be the cause of the weakening periodontal ligament collagen fibers.

"Collagen is the primary connective tissue fiber in the gingiva and periodontal ligament, and the major organic constituent of supporting alveolar bone. In addition, it is the principal component of the sulcular epithelial basement membrane, and thus plays a vital role in promoting the protective barrier function. Collagen within the gingival tissue has a high turnover rate; therefore, it has been postulated that the actual optimal ascorbate requirements of the gingiva may be greater than what can be supplied by ingesting the recommended daily allowance."(4)

Although it is one of the most researched vitamins in the world, scientists and researchers are still discovering new and important metabolic aspects of vitamin C in humans. It is necessary for the synthesis of collagen; the absorption of dietary iron; and is essential for the maintenance of the adrenal cortex. It functions as a strong antioxidant helping to control free radicals as well as working synergistically with vitamins A and E. It is necessary for the metabolism of some important amino acids and the formation of cartilage, dentine, and bone; and the maintenance of healthy capillaries.

It also has some identified relationships with heart disease and stroke. "A 20-year follow-up study suggested that higher levels of intake of vitamin C correlated closely with a reduced risk of death from stroke and this association was strongly related with death as diastolic blood pressure."(5) "Thirty days of oral treatment with vitamin C improves endothelium-dependent vasodilation in patients with coronary artery disease, and even a single dose of 2 grams can improve vasomotor function after 2 hours."(5)

In today's stressful fast paced life, we believe it is essential that everyone supplement with vitamin C.

Oral Health and Heart Disease

Coenzyme Q10 (CoQ10)

Most people in this country are not too familiar with CoQ10. However, it has been used for years in Japan and Europe. What is so appropriate about taking CoQ10 for periodontal disease is that there are hundreds of studies demonstrating its effectiveness in cardiovascular disease.

Every cell in our body contains organelles called mitochondria, where energy in the form of adenosine triphosphate (ATP) is produced. ATP is directly responsible for all energy production at the cellular level and is therefore essential to cellular health and function. Although CoQ10 is synthesized within our bodies, our internal ability to supply Co10 declines with increasing age, malnourishment or chronic illness.

CoQ10 in periodontal disease.

The specific activity of a CoQ10 enzyme was determined in a group of 29 periodontal patients. All 29 patients showed a deficiency of CoQ10-enzyme activity in gingival biopsies. In corresponding blood samples from these patients, 86% showed deficiencies of 20-66% and higher. Periodontal patients frequently have significant gingival and leucocytic (white blood cell) deficiencies of CoQ10, which indicates a systemic nutritional imbalance and is not likely caused by neglected oral hygiene. A gingival deficiency could predispose this tissue to periodontitis and this disease could even aggravate the deficiency.(6)

COMMENT: It would appear that if CoQ10 diminishes as we age, or suffer from malnutrition or chronic illness, deficiencies of CoQ10 in oral tissues could also be a positive warning sign indicating total body deficiencies of this critical nutrient, which is necessary for human life.

In a double-blind study, patients with periodontal disease were treated with 50 mg of CoQ10 per day for three weeks or a matching placebo. Significant results were demonstrated in the patients receiving CoQ10.(7) CoQ10 is fat soluble, meaning that it requires fat to be present for proper assimilation. Many different manufacturers are now providing softgel capsules containing CoQ10 and oil. The Japanese have long used CoQ10 as a therapy to treat gingivitis. In a recent study topical application of CoQ10 to the periodontal pocket was evaluated with and without mechanical root planing and subgingival scaling. In the first 3 weeks of the study only CoQ10 was applied to the pockets and significant reductions in gingival crevicular fluid flow, probing depth and attachment loss were found. After root planing and subgingival debridement significant decreases in the

Oral Health and Heart Disease

plaque index, gingival crevicular fluid flow, probing depth and attachment loss were found both at the experimental and control sites. However, significant improvement in the modified gingival index, bleeding on probing and peptidase activity from periodontopathic bacteria were only observed in the experimental sites where CoQ10 had been applied. These results suggest that topical application of CoQ10 improves adult periodontitis not only as a sole treatment but also in combination with traditional nonsurgical periodontal therapy.(8)

A case history study of a 25-year old male who had such severe and chronic periodontal disease that they were going to extract all teeth, was first treated with hexahydrocoenzyme Q4 which functions like naturally occurring coenzyme Q10 in gingival tissue. After three weeks of treatment an examination revealed initial benefits of the treatment. During the fourth and fifth examinations after the seventh and eighth weeks of treatment, three dentists, separately and independently scored clinically significant improvements of five periodontal disease symptoms. The authors concluded that coenzyme Q could be an important therapeutic adjunct to periodontal therapy for certain patients.(9)

As our immune systems are very much involved in all aspects of our health, including periodontal disease, we thought this next study was extremely important. "Coenzyme Q10 (CoQ10) and vitamin B6 (pyridoxine) have been administered together and separately to three groups of human subjects. The blood levels of CoQ10 increased significantly when CoQ10 and pyridoxine were administered together and when CoQ10 was given alone. The blood levels of IgG (one of five classes of immunoglobulin that function as antibodies in the immune system) increased more significantly when CoQ10 and pyridoxine were given together than when CoQ10 was given alone. The blood levels of T4-lymphocytes (involved in cellular immunity) increased when administered together or separately. The ratio of T4/T8 lymphocytes increased (T8 cells function as killer and suppressor cells in the immune system) more significantly when CoQ10 and pyridoxine were given together than when given separately. The study concluded: "These increases in IgG and T4-lymphocytes with CoQ10 and vitamin B6 are clinically important for trials on AIDS, other infectious diseases, and on cancer."(10)

Cardiovascular disease.

Perhaps the most acclaimed usage of CoQ10 is for cardiovascular disease, since the heart muscle has the highest concentration of CoQ10 in the body. Consequently it is one of the most frequently prescribed heart "drugs" in Japan and is also widely used in Europe. Heart patients have already taken millions of dosages with virtually no serious side effects. In toxicology tests involving thousands of human subjects, no toxicity has ever been observed involving CoQ10. Unlike a drug being administered into the body, CoQ10 is completely natural and is not a substance alien to the human biological system.

The following was a major long-term study on the effectiveness of the use of CoQ10 in clinical cardiology. Although CoQ10 has been found to be non-toxic except in cases of allergic reaction, we think it is important for heart patients to discuss with their physician, before adding CoQ10 to their therapeutic regimen.

Over an eight year period (1985-1993), 424 patients with various forms of cardiovascular disease had CoQ10 added to their medical regimens. Doses of CoQ10 ranged from 75 to 600 mg/day by mouth. Patients were followed for an average of 17.8 months, with a total accumulation of 632 patient years of experience. A statistically significant improvement in myocardial function was documented. Furthermore, before treatment with CoQ10, most patients were taking from one to five cardiac medications. During this study, overall medication requirements dropped considerably: 43% stopped between one and three drugs. Only 6% required the addition of one drug. No apparent side effects from CoQ10 treatment were noted other than a single case of transient nausea. The authors concluded: "CoQ10 is a safe and effective adjunctive treatment for a broad range of cardiovascular diseases, producing gratifying clinical responses while easing the medical and financial burden of multidrug therapy."(11)

"Patients with heart failure have lower levels of myocardial coenzyme Q10 compared with controls. Low plasma coenzyme Q10 levels are associated with an increased mortality in heart failure."(5)

Magnesium.

Here again, we have a double edged nutrient. It is critically important for your heart and there is limited evidence demonstrating it is also important for good oral health. Consequently, deficiencies that effect your teeth and gums may also affect your heart and the reverse is also probably true. If you have heart disease, in all probability you also have periodontal disease. Unfortunately, although there are thousands of research studies on magnesium, there are very few dealing with magnesium and periodontal disease.

Oral Health and Heart Disease

Magnesium is involved metabolically in over three hundred different enzyme systems in the body. It is also important in the metabolism of calcium, potassium, phosphorus, zinc, copper, iron, sodium, cadmium, acetylcholine and nitric oxide. It is also involved in the activation of thiamine and therefore, for a wide variety of crucial body functions. Most people do not get enough magnesium from their food and in balance studies (how much was ingested, absorbed and excreted) they found there was an average deficit of 200 mg of magnesium per day between what is required and what was actually available to the body. An additional problem is that magnesium absorption requires plenty of magnesium in the diet plus, selenium, parathyroid hormone, and vitamins B6 and D. It is apparent using these parameters that magnesium deficiency is probably grossly under reported.

In a recent Russian study, clinical examination of 226 patients with periodontitis revealed that 61% of them had hyperesthesia (increased sensitivity, particularly a painful sensation from a normally painless touch stimulus) of the hard dental tissues, characterized by a marked reaction to thermal, chemical and tactile stimulants. Evaluation of biopsy specimens from bone tissue and gingival fluid demonstrated decreasing levels of magnesium, calcium and phosphorus. The combination of clinical manifestations of periodontitis and hyperesthesia necessitate a search for a combined therapy aimed at simultaneous elimination of hyperesthesia and inflammation. (12)

A 1999 Russian study tested a product called Polycatane on patients with periodontal disease. Polycatane (contains bischofite, a mineral containing up to 95% dry residue of magnesium chloride) was effective in the treatment of patients with chronic catarral gingivitis and generalized periodontitis of light and medium severity.(13)

Another study analyzed tissue mineral differences between roots of periodontally diseased teeth in comparison to roots from normal teeth. Minerals consistently found were phosphorus, calcium, copper, zinc, magnesium and sodium. They were in similar concentrations throughout the area analyzed. Magnesium and copper values were higher in nondiseased teeth and there were no differences in concentrations for calcium, phosphorus, zinc and sodium between roots exposed to a periodontal pocket and nondiseased roots.(14)

In an animal study magnesium deficiency was induced to determine if it caused bone loss. The data indicated that magnesium depletion in the rat altered bone and mineral metabolism resulting in bone loss.(15)

Oral Health and Heart Disease

Before we go any further, we want to provide you with a definition of dental calculus: "a hard, stonelike concretion, varying in color from creamy yellow to black, that forms on the teeth or dental prostheses through **calcification** of dental plaque. According to location, there are two general types: supragingival calculus and *subgingival calculus*."(Dorland's Medical Dictionary)

Calculus occurs in many forms in the body. Kidney stones for example are also called calculus, although there is a different mineral composition. Consequently, we wanted to bring out the fact that magnesium has been used successfully to reduce or eliminate the formation of kidney stones. Is it directly applicable to dental calculus? We don't know because research has not been done in this area.

"Magnesium is a known inhibitor of the formation of calcium oxalate crystals in the urine and was proposed for prophylactic treatment in renal stone disease as early as the 17th and 18th centuries."(16) This study involved 55 patients who were being treated on an outpatient basis for recurrent renal calcium stone disease. None of the patients were magnesium deficient. Treatment required each patient to take 500 mg of magnesium daily. The mean stone episode rate decreased from 0.8 to 0.08 stones per year on treatment and 85% of the patients remained free of recurrence during follow-up, whereas 59% of the patients in the control group (no magnesium supplementation) continued their stone formation.(16)

In another study recurrent kidney stone formers were given a combined supplement of magnesium oxide (300 mg/day) and vitamin B6 (10 mg/day) to see its biochemical effect. Serum magnesium significantly increased after 30 days of treatment and the urinary excretion of calcium oxalate (the major component of kidney stones) decreased. What this means is that the patients in the study were not forming as much calcium oxalate and as a result, their risk index for forming stones decreased significantly.(17)

Serum magnesium is a poor indicator of actual magnesium status. A better indicator of the true magnesium status of the body is intracellular red blood cell magnesium levels. We are also aware of some physicians using a new test that does not require giving a blood sample but merely uses a gentle scraping of the oral mucosa to achieve the same results. Should you be taking magnesium? Whether you have periodontal disease or not we believe that everyone should be taking a magnesium supplement. For individuals with periodontal disease we feel it is essential to supplement with magnesium and vitamin B6.

Oral Health and Heart Disease

It is truly unfortunate that so little research has been done on magnesium and oral health. It's a different story regarding the use of magnesium in cardiovascular diseases. There are thousands of research studies addressing the use of magnesium in almost every aspect of heart disease, from the amount in drinking water to intravenous use in emergency medicine to treat myocardial infarction. It is hard to believe that in the year 2001 that there is so much controversy concerning the therapeutic use of magnesium in medicine. The biggest controversy relates to its intravenous use in emergency room settings. Our concern deals with the use of diet and oral supplements to maintain intracellular magnesium levels and the prevention of hypomagnesium.

Magnesium is the second most abundant intracellular cation and is critically involved in energy metabolism and protein and nucleic acid synthesis. "Approximately half of the total magnesium in the body is present in soft tissue, and the other half in bone. Less than 1% of the total body magnesium is present in blood. Nonetheless, the majority of our experimental information comes from determination of magnesium in serum and red blood cells."(18) (Which, do not necessarily correlate with intracellular magnesium.) "As some indication of its broad effect, magnesium deficiency can cause weakness, tremors, seizures, cardiac arrhythmia, low potassium, and low calcium. A large segment of the U.S. population may have an inadequate intake of magnesium and may have a chronic latent magnesium deficiency that has been linked to atherosclerosis, myocardial infarction, hypertension, cancer, kidney stones, premenstrual syndrome, and psychiatric disorders."(18)

Without inundating you with a great number of studies, we would like to highlight a few: "Perioperative use of magnesium can reduce the incidence of arrhythmic events on the atrial and ventricular level. Oral magnesium has been used for many years in patients with symptomatic extrasystoles. Studies show that the incidence of extrasystoles as well as patients' symptoms are reduced during oral magnesium therapy.(19) Patients with idiopathic mitral valve prolapse who were suffering from magnesium deficiency were given 3000 mg a day of magnesium orotate (500 mg tablets) for 6 months. The therapy completely or partially reduced the symptoms in more than half the patients.(20) In a randomized, double-blind, placebo-controlled trial, patients with coronary artery disease (CAD) were given magnesium or a placebo. After 6 months of therapy the study conclusion was: "Oral magnesium therapy in CAD patients is associated with significant improvement in brachial artery endothelial function and exercise tolerance, suggesting a potential mechanism by which magnesium could beneficially alter outcomes in ability to perform.(24) The amino acid methionine plays a critical role in the transsulfuration pathways of the body. During normal metabolism, methionine is partially converted to homocysteine, a toxic amino acid. Homocysteine is also partially converted back to methionine and other non-toxic amino acids. If this process doesn't work efficiently, homocysteine builds up in bodily fluids and tissues, causing undesirable physiological problems.(25)

Vitamin B6 is required for these metabolic changes to occur as is folic acid and vitamin B12, especially in the case of homocysteine. Mercury can disrupt this metabolic process in two ways, first it can bind with the thiol (sulfur) groups in methionine reducing its availability and second it can diminish the effectiveness of vitamin B6. The result of these modifications of metabolism is the unwanted build up of homocysteine. Currently scientists are focusing more and more on the fact that high homocysteine levels can cause serious heart problems.

Like any other new risk factor for cardiovascular disease, there is a great deal of controversy within the medical and scientific communities concerning the true impact of homocysteine on heart disease. There are many studies claiming it is not a risk factor and a greater number of studies indicating that it is. The very fact that the potential exists is reason enough to take protective action. Although no research has as yet been done proving the hypothesis, it would seem reasonable to believe that if you have periodontal disease and amalgam fillings, then you are going to have higher than normal levels of homocysteine.

In addition to anything else you are doing to correct your periodontal problems, you should be supplementing with extra methionine and vitamin B6 to overcome the deficiencies caused by mercury. At the same time, you should insure that you are taking extra supplements of folic acid and vitamin B12 which are also factors in the metabolism of homocysteine.

Vitamin E

Vitamin E functions as a potent antioxidant to protect vitamin A, the carotenes, and unsaturated fatty acids from destructive oxidation. A great deal of recent research has focused on free radicals, reactive oxygen species and antioxidant defense mechanisms. As periodontal disease is a tissue inflammatory disease both free radicals and reactive oxygen species are involved.

In this context, vitamin E as an antioxidant should have a therapeutic effect on periodontal inflammation. "There is evidence that vitamin E increases cell membrane resistance to oxidative destruction and inhibits prostaglaㅡsis. These latter two properties can theoretically increase host resist periodontium to inflammatory-mediated tissue destruction."(26) In ㅡnal study, the animals were given a gingivectomy and half were put on vitamin E (60 I.U. daily) and the other half did not receive any supplementation of vitamin E. The animals receiving the vitamin E supplements healed more rapidly, with almost complete restoration of gingiva by 7 days.(27)

In another animal study, the effect of vitamin E supplementation on alveolar bone loss was studied. Two groups of rats were either stressed or not stressed on a rotational device for 90 days. Vitamin E had a significant protective effect which was most pronounced at sites most susceptible to loss. Stressed subjects tended to lose more bone, but this effect was not significant. These findings suggest some role for vitamin E supplementation in the maintenance of periodontal health but also a sensitivity in this effect to initial periodontal status.(28)

In a Russian study on patients with periodontitis, application of antioxidant vitamin therapy using vitamins A, E and K locally and taking them orally normalized the parameters being considered in this particular study and improved the status of the periodontium.(29)

"High vitamin E intake is associated with a lower incidence of coronary heart disease in middle-aged subjects."(5) "The men in the top 20% of vitamin intake had a 40% lower risk of developing coronary artery disease and in women a 34% risk reduction was seen."(5) "Similar results are seen in those 65 years old and older with additional benefits if subjects took both vitamin E and vitamin C supplements."(5)

Folic Acid

Folacin is a generic term used to describe folic acid and related compounds which exhibit the biological activity of folic acid. Traditionally, most people associate vitamin B12 with folic acid and a great many supplement manufacturers make products that combine both folic acid and vitamin B12. The reason for this is the fact that if you only supplemented with folic acid, the potential exists to mask a deficiency of vitamin B12. This is why the FDA has set a requirement that supplements cannot contain more than 800 mcg of folic acid and higher potencies can only be obtained by doctors prescription. In addition to its synergy with vitamin B12, folic acid works synergistically with biotin, pantothenic acid, niacin, vitamins B1, B2, B6, and C, iron, copper, estradiol, and testosterone. Its basic function is to transfer one carbon units in the metabolism of amino acids.(30, 31)

Deficiencies of folic acid are pretty wide spread because it is easily destroyed by cooking or food processing. Compounding this problem is the fact that anticonvulsants, alcohol, and oral contraceptives produce low serum and tissue concentrations of folate. Signs and symptoms of folate deficiency might include anemia, fatigue, irritability, peripheral neuropathy, diarrhea, weight loss, and gingivitis. A decrease of folic acid in the gingiva leads to a decrease in resistance of the gingiva to local irritants resulting in an increase in inflammation.(32)

Previously we outlined how a folate mouthwash was effective in reducing gingivitis, so it appears that both oral supplementation and topical application are effective in reducing gingival inflammation as determined by decreased redness, bleeding, tenderness, exudate, and plaque scores.(17,18,32)

Folic acid is another nutrient that has a very special role in cardiovascular disease. Several studies utilizing folic acid alone, or in conjunction with vitamins B6, B12 and betaine (trimethylglycine) have demonstrated the ability of these nutrients to normalize homocysteine levels. As pointed out earlier, high levels of homocysteine are now being considered as an important risk factor in the development of heart disease.

Thiamine (Vitamin B1)

It is commonly believed that a deficiency of thiamine rarely occurs. That may have been true at one time, but it certainly isn't true today given the average lifestyle in industrialized countries, especially in the United states. Thiamine plays a very key roll in the metabolism of carbohydrates, and is essential in nerve biochemistry. Therefore, if one looks at the average diet from childhood into adulthood it is obvious that there is an inordinate consumption of sugar, white refined flour breads, pastries, cakes etc., "soft" drinks containing sugar and caffeine, fruit drinks, alcohol, candy bars and confections most of which contain high levels of sugar, etc. These types of food all generate "naked" calories and thiamine requirements are dependent upon calories ingested. Consequently, excessive consumption of carbohydrates, and inadequate intake of thiamine can be considered primary causative factors leading to a chronic deficiency of thiamine. Peer pressures, stress, alcohol consumption, and a variety of pharma-

Oral Health and Heart Disease

ceuticals, including diuretics (a common prescription for anyone with cardiovascular disease and especially the elderly), and a number of antibiotics all contribute to the chronic thiamine deficiency state.

There is another aspect of induced thiamine deficiency that has not been addressed. Vitamin B1 is one of only two vitamins that have a sulfur component (the other is biotin). Because of its sulfur moiety we hypothesize that mercury will bind to thiamine making it unavailable for its normal metabolic functions and at the same time augmenting any deficiency state. Therefore, if you have amalgam dental fillings, the mercury being continuously released and migrating into the mucosa and alveolar bone, has the potential to create or greatly exacerbate a thiamine deficiency in the periodontium.

Thiamine (vitamin B1) deficiency is characterized by polyneuritis (inflammation of several peripheral nerves at once), cardiac pathology and edema. Beri-beri is a thiamine deficiency disease. There are two forms, dry and wet. Dry beri-beri involves muscular atrophy, an absence of reflexes (areflexia), cardiac enlargement, and tachycardia may also be present. Wet beri-beri is a form marked by cardiac failure and edema, but without extensive nervous system involvement. (Dorland's Medical Dictionary)

"Thiamine deficiency can induce high-output cardiac failure due to the accumulation of pyruvate and lactate, leading to intense vasodilation. Response to thiamine is brisk and often with full recovery."(5) "Frusemide-induced thiamine deficiency was first described in rats and thiamine uptake by cardiac myocytes is significantly impaired both by digoxin and frusemide, the drugs having an additive effect if given together."(5) "Thiamine supplementation in patients with moderate-to-severe congestive heart failure(CHF) taking 80 mg of frusemide induced a significant improvement in left ventricular ejection fraction and symptoms."(5) (frusemide and digoxin are heart medications)

It is obvious that a deficiency of thiamine is involved in maintaining a healthy heart but where and how does it become involved in oral health? In 1953, the results of a comprehensive study on the therapeutic use of thiamine in dentistry was published in the U.S. Armed Forces Medical Journal. The study has never been replicated, nor has anyone ever followed up on the dramatic information contained therein. The study was done by a military dentist, James L.E. Bock, Lt. Col, USAF at the Bolling Air Force Base Dental Clinic in Washington, D.C. and encompassed hundreds of clinic patients. The purpose of the study was to evaluate the use of thiamine injections to treat various oral diseases or conditions. In

Oral Health and Heart Disease

conjunction with the clinical aspects, Dr. Bock did a very extensive literature research on every aspect of the conditions he was going to treat with thiamine. The study was so comprehensive that it was published in three parts in three different issues of the Journal. For those of you who might be interested in reviewing this study, we have published a book on Vitamin B1 which includes all three parts of Col. Bock's study. It can be purchased by calling Bio-Probe at 1-800-282-9670.

Dental caries

"Various theories have been advanced for the cause of dental caries. One cause that has been suggested is malnutrition. Thiamine deficiency has been singled out as one factor in malnutrition which may affect dental caries by producing an acid saliva."(33) A supporting study by Hearman, suggested that in the absence of thiamine, the normal breakdown of pyruvate, formed during carbohydrate fermentation, does not occur and acid, which results in decalcification at the gingival margins, is liberated.(34) Although subsequent studies by other authors produced differing results, there have been recent studies that tend to support Hearman. A recent case history, of an individual who was admitted to the hospital with metabolic acidosis and heart failure, was treated with IV thiamine which resulted in a dramatic clearing of both conditions.(35) . A French article just published, discussed "Shoshin", a fulminating form of cardiac beri-beri that without specific treatment progresses rapidly towards cardiogenic shock and metabolic acidosis The authors stated that treatment with thiamine and alkalinization permits a spectacular and fast recovery.(36) A dietary evaluation of Finnish children with high caries experience revealed that the diets of this group contained less thiamine, ascorbic acid and iron.(37) If you are prone to caries and your saliva pH is in the acidic range, a simple method of evaluating the efficacy of vitamin B1 would be to take your saliva pH, supplement with 100 mg of Vitamin B1, and a couple of hours later take your saliva pH again and see if it moved from acid towards alkaline.

Treatment of dental pain

Where thiamine really shines is in its therapeutic use in controlling dental pain. Nerve cells require vitamin B1 in order to function properly and deficiencies of this nutrient can effect the peripheral nervous system. Dr. Bock successfully treated a number of dental disorders using either thiamine injections or by infiltrating thiamine directly into the gum tissue.

Oral Health and Heart Disease

Patients deficient in thiamine show a marked sensitivity of the oral tissues (38) and extreme sensitiveness of the teeth to instrumentation and an abnormal thermal response.(39) Dr. Bock treated a substantial number of his patients with hypersensitive teeth or pain related to other dental disorders such as trauma following operation, deep scaling, overhanging fillings, ill-fitting partial dentures, fractures, traumatic occlusion, deep fillings, Vincent's infection, gingivitis associated with pregnancy, with 100 mg of thiamine hydrochloride injected intramuscularly daily until symptoms were relieved. In most patients one injection was sufficient. Beneficial results were obtained in from 20 to 30 minutes.(33) He also used intraoral injections of 10 mg of thiamine hydrochloride infiltrated directly into the submucosa to relieve the pain of hypersensitive teeth or of pain associated with operative procedures such as gingivectomy. In most patients complete relief of pain was obtained within ten minutes of receiving the thiamine injection.(33)

Unfortunately, most dentists have never heard of using thiamine injections for the relief of pain. Consequently, it is a treatment modality that is just not available. The standard of care for pain is to prescribe non-steroidal drugs (NSAIDs), or if severe, to prescribe narcotics. Fortunately, however, Dr. Bock and other researchers did some experimentation using oral doses of vitamin B1 to control pain. What is so amazing about these endeavors is that the highest dosage used in most cases did not exceed 10 mg of Vitamin B1.

For example, in the case of herpes simplex and herpes zoster, Dr. Bock reported that these conditions had been successfully treated with oral doses of thiamine hydrochloride (vitamin B1). "Burket and Hickman (40) reported 6 patients with herpes simplex, 3 of whom were treated with thiamine hydrochloride and vitamin B complex and 3 with thiamine hydrochloride alone. The oral administration of 5 mg in a patient with recurrent herpetic lesions resulted in complete resolution. A solitary aphthous lesion was treated with 3 mg of thiamine daily with complete disappearance in 48 hours. Aphthous lesions appeared in one patient every time walnuts were eaten. This patient was cleared of the lesions with 3 mg of thiamine orally within 48 hours. When the same dose was used as a prophylactic measure, aphthous lesions failed to appear after the patient ate walnuts."(33)

"Herpes zoster affects the spinal and cranial nerves. The first division of the trigeminal nerve is most frequently involved. (41) Ratner and Roll (42) reported 16 patients with herpes zoster treated with vitamin B1, of whom 5 were relieved of pain and 11 were not." They used doses of 3 to 6 mg daily. Waldman and

Oral Health and Heart Disease

Pelner (43), using 100 mg of thiamine intramuscularly, were more successful. Relief of pain was obtained in 23 patients with from 2 to 6 injections.

There are many different factors that we believe affect the amount of thiamine the body will absorb out of the gut. In an ideal healthy person, the absorption would be very low. However, as exertion, infection, inflammation and pain all increase the need for thiamine, the absorption of oral supplementation of thiamine increases to meet the need. We were able to find a paper published in 1986 that sheds light on the subject of thiamine absorption. *H.Quirin* discussed a German study done by *Bötticher* et al.utilizing a new analytical method (high-performance liquid chromatogaraphy) that demonstrated that progressively higher doses (up to 4 g/day) of orally administered thiamine increased thiamine blood concentrations. (44)

Based on *Böttcher's* findings, *Quirin* treated 133 patients suffering from headache and diverse forms of arthralgia, spinal syndromes, and neuralgia. All had previously been treated with physical therapy or analgesic drugs without benefit. Physical therapy was continued but a dose of 1-2 grams of thiamine (500 mg tablets) was added and was repeated 1-2 times per day. Out of the 133 patients, 99 (73%) showed satisfactory or very good results in relieving pain.(44)

A recent double-blind study involving 556 girls aged 12-21 years with moderate to very severe spasmodic dysmenorrhoea (painful menstruation) evaluated its efficacy in relieving pain. A daily dose of 100 mg of vitamin B1 was given orally for 90 days; 87 percent of the study patients were completely cured and in 8 percent the pain was reduced significantly, while 5 percent of the patients showed no effect whatsoever. The results remained the same two months later without any further supplementation of vitamin B1.(45)

Long before I ever read Dr. Bock's article I was using vitamin B1 supplements to control pain associated with any dental visit. I would take 200 mg of vitamin B1 and 200 mg of vitamin B6 (to control swelling and trauma) 30 minutes before my appointment and take the same amount after completion of the dental work. I never needed to take any medication for pain or swelling, even if surgery was involved. Interestingly, in a study involving 200 diabetic patients with peripheral neuropathy the worst symptoms of which were pain, numbness and paraesthesia, were treated with 25 mg of vitamin B1 and 50 mg of vitamin B6 a day for four weeks. At the end of that time the severity of signs of peripheral neuropathy had decreased 48.9%.(46)

Oral Health and Heart Disease

Further research attempting to determine if vitamin B6 also had analgesic properties revealed that in addition to its ability to limit swelling, vitamin B6 plays an essential role in tryptophan metabolism. Further, serotonin formation from tryptophan is directly dependent on vitamin B6 and it also plays a role in the biosynthesis of dopamine. In animal experiments, vitamin B6 has shown a central analgesic effect.(47)

This study also revealed significant information about the ability of vitamin C, vitamin K, and vitamin B12 to also effectively reduce pain. High dose vitamin C was shown to be very effective for the relief of pain in a variety of diseases and conditions including bone pain of Paget's disease, reduction of pain related to the lumbar disk, from bone metastases, and in cancer patients either alone or together with a drug analgesic (when the drug had become ineffective in stopping the pain). Further, the combination of vitamin B1, B6, B12 taken together showed an excellent effect, dose-dependent and comparable to phenylbutaxone (a drug with analgesic, antipyretic, anti-inflammatory properties) in both the therapeutic anti-inflammatory and in the analgesic test.(47) The highest dose used in the previous experiment was 20 mg B1, 20 mg B6, and 0.24 mg B12.

All of the studies cited above, whether human or animal, utilized small doses of the particular vitamins being tested. The patients involved were all suffering with symptoms that certainly must have depleted their body stores of vitamin B1, B6, B12, and C. Would 100 mg a day of vitamin B1, or B6, or B12 or 3000 mg a day of vitamin C have helped a greater number of patients in a shorter period of time is a legitimate question that science should answer? The vitamins in question are all inexpensive, non-toxic and water soluble, meaning that any excess dosage over and above what the body needs is going to be excreted, so why worry about how low a dose will help a particular condition. You are a special and uniquely biochemical individual and there are no tests or standards to let you know how much of a particular nutrient your body may need biochemically when being stressed by chronic or acute pain. Consequently, the penalty you pay for erring on the high side is a urine rich in vitamin metabolic by-products. A price most individuals would willingly pay to relieve their pain.

Manufactured Periodontol Formulas

As stated in an earlier disclaimer, we are not recommending or advocating the use of any particular product. Our intent is to provide relevant information of use

Oral Health and Heart Disease

to patients and health care providers. In this context, we think it extremely important to tell you about one company that in our opinion has truly done something important in the use of nutritional supplementation to treat periodontal disease. The company is called "Pharmaden" and after years of research, they have formulated and produced a group of products designed solely to provide nutritional support for patients with periodontal problems. The products can only be purchased through a dentist who essentially subscribes to and believes in nutritional support as an adjunct to periodontal treatment. Ethical considerations would not permit a dentist selling you the products unless you were under his or her care for treatment of your periodontal problem. You can call 1-800-910-5523 to find a dentist near you who uses *Pharmaden* products in treating periodontal disease, or you can ask your own dentist to call and get an informational packet complete with scientific justification for their adjunctive use in any periodontal treatment protocol. *Pharmaden* manufactures four different products that cover initial treatment, post treatment support, special formulations for addressing bone loss and surgical periodontal treatment. Loma Linda University recently completed a double-blind study on *Pharmaden's* PerioTherapy™ which demonstrated a significant reduction in pocket depth, bleeding index, and gingival index.(48)

Oral Health and Heart Disease

References

1. Cherasskin E. and Ringsdorf WM., Jr. Effect of regular versus sustained-release multivitamin supplementation upon periodontal parameters: II Sulcus depth and clinical tooth mobility. Internat. J Vit Res 1969;39:476-485.
2. Ziff S, Ziff MF. Simplified Guide to Nutritional Supplements. Bio-Probe, Inc, Orlando, FL, 1994 pp 29.
3. Jacob RA, et al. Experimental vitamin C depletion and supplementation in young men. Nutrient interactions and dental health effects. Ann N Y Sci 1987;498L333-346.
4. Pollack RL, Kravitz E. Nutrition in Oral Health and Disease. Lea & Febiger, Philadelphia, pp 141-142, 174-175, 207, 407, 1985.
5. Klaus K., et al. Chronic Heart Failure and Micronutrients. J Am Coll Cardiol 2001;37:1765-1774.
6. Hansen IL., et al. Bioenergetics in clinical medicine. IX. Gingival and leucocytic deficiencies of coenzyme Q10 in patients with periodontal disease. Res Commun Chem Pathol Pharmacol 1976 Aug;14(4):729-738.
7. Wilkinson EG, Arnold RM, Folkers K. Bioenergetics in clinical medicine. VI. adjunctive treatment of periodontal disease with coenzyme Q10. Res Commun Chem Pathol Pharmacol 1976 Aug;14(4):715-719.
8. Hajioka T., et al. Effect of topical application of coenzyme Q10 on adult periodontitis. Mol Aspects Med 1994;15 Suppl:s241-248.
9. Iwamoto Y, Nakamura R, Folkers K, Morrison RF. Study of periodontal disease and coenzyme Q. Res Commun Chem Pathol Pharmacol 1975 Jun; 11(2):265-271.
10. Folkers K, Morita M, McRee J Jr. The activities of coenzyme Q10 and vitamin B6 for immune responses. Biochem Biophys Res Commun 1993 May 28;193(1):88-92.
11. Langsjoen H., et al. Usefulness of coenzyme Q10 in clinical cardiology: a long-term study. Mol Aspects Med 1994;15 Suppl:s165-175.
12. Beloklitskaia GF. Indices characterizing the expression of hyperesthesia of the hard dental tissues in patients with periodontitis. Stomatologiia (Mosk) 1992 Jan-Feb;(1):29-31 (article in Russian)
13. Spasov AA., et al. The experimental and clinical validation of the use of a polikatan preparation in periodontal disease. Stomatologiia (Mosk) 1999:78(5):16-19. (In Russian)
14. Barton NS, Van Swol RL. Periodontally diseased vs. normal roots as evaluated by scanning electron microscopy and electron probe analysis. J Periodontol 1987 Sep;58(9):634-638..
15. Rude RK., et al. Magnesium deficiency induces bone loss in the rat. Miner Electrolyte Metab 1998;24(5):314-320.

Oral Health and Heart Disease

16. Johansson G., et al. Effects of magnesium hydroxide in renal stone disease. J Am Coll Nutr 1982:1(2):179-185.
17. Rattan V., et al. Effect of combined supplementation of magnesium oxide and pyridoxine in calcium-oxalate stone formers. Urol Res 1994;22(3):161-165.
18. Elin RJ. Magnesium metabolism in health and disease. Dis Mon 1988 Apr;34(4):161-218.
19. Stublinger HG, Kiss K, Smetana R. Significance of magnesium in cardiac arrhythmiaas. Wien Med Wochenschr 2000;150(15-16):330-334.(Article in German)
20. Martynov AI., et al. New approaches to the treatment of patients with idiopathic mitral valve prolapse. Ter Arkh 2000;72(9):67-70. (In Russian)
21. Shechter M., et al. Oral magnesium therapy improves endothelial function in patients with coronary artery disease. Circulation 2000 Nov 7;102(19):2353-2358
22. Shechter M. et al. Low intracellular magnesium levels promote platelet-dependent thrombosis in patients with coronary artery disease. Am Heart J 2000 Aug;140(2):212-218.
23. Sueda S. et al. Magnesium deficiency in patients with recent myocardial infarction and provoked coronary artery spasm. Jpn Circ J 2001 Jul;65(7):643-648.
24. Liu Y., et al. The mechanism of Hg2+ toxicity in cultured human oral fibroblasts: the involvement of cellular thiols. Chem Biol Interact 1992 Nov 30;85(1):69-78.
25. Frankel P, Kim C. Beyond AntiOxidants Methylation Homocysteine and Nutrition. The Research Corner, 1996
26. Robert L Pollack, Edward Kravitz. Nutrition in Oral Health and Disease. 1985;pp138.Lea & Febiger, Philadelphia.
27. Kim JF, Snklar G. The effect of vitamin E on the healing of gingival wounds in rats. J Periodontol 1983 May;54(5):305-308.
28. Cohen ME, Meyer DM. Effect of dietary vitamin E supplementation and rotational stress on alveolar bone loss in rice rats. Arch Oral Biol 1993 Jul;38(7):601-606.
29. Khmelevskii IV., et al. Effect of vitamins A, E, and K on the indicies of the glutathione antiperoxide system in gingival tissues in periodontosis. Vopr Pitan 1985 Jul-Aug;(4):54-56.
30. Nutrition Review. Present Knowledge in Nutrition (Fifth Edition) The Nutrition Foundation, Inc., Washington, D.C., 1984:332-346.
31. Kutsky RJ. Handbook of Vitamins, Minerals and Hormones (2nd Edition) Van Nostrand Reinhold Co., New York, NY. 1981:269-277.
32. Kelly GS. Folates: supplemental forms and therapeutic applications. Altern Med Rev 1998 Jun;3(3):208-220.
33. Ziff S, Ziff M. Vitamin B1 for Dentistry! Medicine! Research! Bio-Probe, Inc. Orlando, Fl, 1996.
34. Hearman CD. Digest of etiology of dental caries. Dental J Australia 1939 Nov;11:692.

Oral Health and Heart Disease

35. Ozawa H. et al. Severe metabolic acidosis and heart failure due to thiamine deficiency. Nutrition 2001 Apr;17(4):351-352.

36. Masset C., Lancellotti P, Nkoghe D. Shoshin beriberi: myth or reality? Rev Med Liege 2001 Mar;56(3):155-158.

37. Kleemola-Kujala E, Rasanen L. Dietary pattern of Finnish children with low high caries experience. Community Dent Oral Epidemiol 1979 Aug; 7(4):199-205.

38. Mann AW; Spies TD and Springer M. Oral manifestations of vitamin B complex deficiencies. J Dent Research 1941;20:269.

39. Sinclair JA. Vitamin A and B deficiency--etiologic factors in acute, subacute and chronic Vincent's infection and other dental conditions. J Am Dent Assoc 1939;26:1611-1618

40. Burket LW and Hickman GC. Oral herpes (simplex) manifestations; treatment with vitamin B complex. J Am Dent Assoc. 1942;29:411-418.

41. Burket LW. Oral Medicine. J.P. Lippincott Co., Philadeplphia, Pa. 1946. pp 152.

42. Rattner H. and Roll HC. Herpes zoster and vitamin B1. JAMA 1939 June 24;112:2585-2586.

43. Waldman S and Pelner L. Treatment of essential (idiopathic) herpes zoster by thiamine potentiated with neostigmine. NY State J Med 1947 Sept 15;47:1997-1999.

44. Quirin H. Pain and Vitamin B1 Therapy. Biblthca Nutr Dieta 1986;38:110-111.

45. Gokhale LB. Curative treatment of primary (spasmodic) dysmenorrhoea. Indian J Med Res 1996 Apr;103:227-231.

46. Abbas ZG, Swai AB. Evaluation of the efficacy of thiamine and pyridoxine in the treatment of symptomatic diabetic peripheral neuropathy. East Afr Med J 1997 Dec;74(12):803-808.

47. Hanck A, Weiser H. Analgesic and anti-inflammatory properties of vitamins. Int J Vitam Nutr Res Suppl 1985;27:189-206.

48. Munoz CA., et al. Effects of a nutritional supplement on periodontal status. Compendium 2001 May;22(5):425-438.

Oral Health and Heart Disease

Chapter 8
Biocompatible Periodontal Therapy (BPT)

The first order of business is to define what conventional periodontal therapy, as taught in dental schools, is and how Biocompatible Periodontal Therapy differs.

Establishment periodontal therapy employs two basic types of therapy identified as nonsurgical and surgical:

Nonsurgical treatment involves scaling with an ultrasonic scaler and instruments to remove plaque and calculus from the teeth that are above the gum line (supragingival). Treatment of deep periodontal pockets below the gum line (subgingival) that do not require any cutting of the gingiva for access, are treated by root planing. This procedure requires either topical or injected anesthesia to permit planing of the entire length of the root. Calling root planing nonsurgical is really a misnomer in that the procedure intended to remove hardened calculus deposits actually, in addition to calculus, removes healthy root structure supposedly as a means of causing subsequent healing. Unfortunately, this procedure can also preclude periodontal re-attachment. However, Loesch in his 1999 paper on the use of antibiotics in periodontal therapy advocated a new paradigm which he calls "The Specific Plaque Hypothesis," intended to treat the bacterial infection with short-term use of antibiotics in conjunction with debridement before any surgical intervention.(1) The rationale being that treatment with antibiotics reduces the cause of periodontal disease, while surgical therapy reduces the result of the periodontal infection. Although the protocol still calls for root planing it appears that it could be considered movement of establishment dentistry towards biocompatible periodontal treatment.

Surgical treatment is just what the term implies. The gums are cut open to permit the periodontist to accomplish root planing or whatever other treatment is planned to treat the periodontal condition..

What separates Biocompatible Periodontal Therapy from that outlined above is the philosophy of eliminating the infection causing periodontal disease without removing healthy tooth structure. I like the terminology used by Corbet and his colleagues in a 1993 study in which he called the subgingival action "bacterial debridement."(2) BPT starts with the premise that the condition is caused by a chronic infection by pathogenic microorganisms that have, in effect, overcome

Oral Health and Heart Disease

your own immune system. Consequently, the most important aspect to therapy is the elimination of the microorganisms causing the problem in the first place, with the intent of accomplishing this hopefully without the use of antibiotics, unless deemed absolutely necessary. The next most important aspect is to provide dietary and nutritional guidance augmenting support for normal immune function to successfully control subsequent microorganism exposures.

This protocol requires that you, as the patient, become an active participant in achieving oral health. The dentist or hygienist cannot do it all. Once they have commenced their treatment plan, you become the most important member of the team. Without you applying the outlined home treatment religiously, **IT IS IMPOSSIBLE TO GET RID OF PERIODONTAL DISEASE.**

Why so much emphasis on the need for oral hygiene away from the dental office? A recent scientific study in Japan clearly answers the question. The study took place over a four year period. Initially, microbiological samples were obtained from three different periodontal sites in each participant. Then, a base line status for each participant was recorded for missing teeth, presence of plaque, gingivitis, probing pocket depth, probing attachment level and gingival recession. For the first two years, patients went without any periodontal treatment. The patients were instructed to just continue their normal oral hygiene routine which, consisted of brushing their teeth twice a day using a toothpaste. Assessment at the end of two years demonstrated that the periodontal condition did not deteriorate further.(3)

At the beginning of the third year 62 patients out of the original 300 in the study were selected to participate in a carefully supervised oral hygiene program. Multitufted soft toothbrushes, interdental brushes and triangular toothpicks were used in the self performed plaque control program. In addition, during the first 3 months the supragingival (above the gum line) portion of the tooth surfaces were carefully instrumented to remove all supragingival plaque and calculus. This instrumentation was performed by 3 operators treating about 20 subjects each. 24 months after starting the supervised home-care program, all subjects were again examined using the same clinical parameters that were taken at the start of the first year. During the first two years, the percentage of plaque harboring tooth surfaces varied between 50 and 60%, while at the end of four years, the mean plaque scores were reduced to about 15%. More importantly, evaluation of the subgingival microbiota indicated a marked reduction in the quantity and composition of subgingival microbiota. The total viable counts of bacteria in both deep

Oral Health and Heart Disease

and shallow pockets were dramatically reduced 2 years after initiation of the enhanced oral hygiene efforts.(3)

This study clearly demonstrated just how important correct and disciplined oral hygiene home-care is to achieving and maintaining good oral health. So, once again without you following the specific instructions given to you by your dentist and hygienist, **IT WILL BE IMPOSSIBLE TO ACHIEVE THE GOAL OF GOOD ORAL HEALTH!**

Some dentists have been practicing various different concepts of biocompatible periodontal therapy for a long time. It appears that the Keyes Technique (early 1970) was the first scientific attempt to correct periodontal disease without surgery. Dr. P. Keyes developed the technique which was based on the microscopic diagnoses of subgingival plaque infections. The Keyes Technique encompassed 1) patient education; 2) oral hygiene with adjunctive antimicrobials (this involved tooth brushing and flossing to remove plaque, supplemented by making a paste of baking soda, hydrogen peroxide, and salt, which was to be worked subgingivally); 3) scaling. 4) microscopic monitoring with a phase contrast microscope (to determine therapeutic effectiveness); antibiotics, if necessary and fluoride gel, if needed. Dr. Keyes also utilized laboratory microbial analysis to determine the appropriate antibiotic if one was required. The Keyes Technique did not fare very well because it was such a radical departure from the existing standard of surgical periodontal treatment.

Dr. Trevor Lyons of Ottawa, Canada, a world class authority on the subject, has long advocated the treatment of the bacterial cause of periodontal disease. In fact, his 1989 book *Introduction to Protozoa and Fungi in Periodontal Infections - A Manual of Microbiological Diagnosis and Nonsurgical Treatment* was one of the catalysts for the International Academy of Oral Medicine and Toxicology (IAOMT) to initiate action to develop and establish BPT as an Approved Standard of Care for IAOMT members. Dr. Thomas E. Baldwin (an avid practitioner of non-surgical periodontal treatment for many years) headed an IAOMT committee that developed the Standard of Care.

The IAOMT is sponsoring teaching seminars on the BPT protocol to be given by Dr. Baldwin and other selected speakers. Dentists who are interested in learning more can contact the IAOMT at 407-298-2450. A great many of the IAOMT dentists are including BPT in their own dental practices. For a referral to an IAOMT dentist near you please call 407-298-2450. However, at the present time there is no specific record of which of the IAOMT members are actively

Oral Health and Heart Disease

employing BPT in their practices. So, once you have the name(s) of dentists you will have to call the their office(s) to find out.

The basic components of BPT are:

Diagnosis:

This involves probing and charting pocket depth; condition of the gingiva; bleeding on probing; odor or purulent discharge; mobility; bone loss and occlusal problems.

Another major element of diagnosis involves microbiological tests. Dentists who are seriously practicing BPT will have a phase contrast microscope in their office. If you have never seen a slide of a sample from an active periodontal site displayed in great magnification on the video screen before your eyes, you are in for a real shocker. It is almost impossible to comprehend how so many different live "creatures" can be present in one tiny sample from a periodontal pocket. You will see a wide range of putative periodontal pathogens, including amoeba and trichomonanads; spirochetes; fungi and yeast. Phase contrast microscopy provides a cost-effective immediate clinical method of diagnosis. Perhaps even more importantly, it provides an exceptionally accurate method of monitoring how much progress is being made in treating the disease.

If a phase contrast microscope is not available, periodontal pocket samples for laboratory analysis will have to be taken and sent to specialized oral microbiology labs, if you are to know what types and quantities of periodontal pathogens with which you are infected. Some of the pathogens in the sample may be fragile and die en route to the lab; however, they can still be identified by DNA analysis to complete the evaluation. If the use of systemic antibiotics is contemplated, this type of culturing and testing is required for the selection of the correct antibiotic. This is true because so many pathogens have developed resistance to so many different antibiotics that it is essential for the testing laboratory to identify which antibiotics will be effective in your individual situation.

The gingival crevice is defined as "a shallow trough or fissure surrounding the anatomic crown of a tooth, considered by some authorities to be the same as the gingival sulcus...called also subgingival

Oral Health and Heart Disease

space." (Dorland's Medical dictionary) An explanation of Gingival Crevicular Fluid (GCF) is provided by a recent article: "The constituents of GCF are derived from a number of sources, including serum, the connective tissue and epithelium through which GCF passes on its way to the crevice, and inflammatory cells and bacteria present in the tissues and crevice."(4)

There is a company, Affinity Labeling Technologies, Inc., that is specializing in providing dentists and physicians with laboratory analytical tests to assist in the identification and diagnosis of infectious oral health problems. One of their products called *TOPAS* (Toxicity Presecreening Assay) provides the dentist with a chair-side test for the detection of bacterial toxins, bacterial proteins and human inflammatory proteins in gingival crevicular fluid (GCF) The *TOPAS* detects 1) increased levels of bacterial toxins and 2) increased levels of human inflammatory and serum proteins as well as bacterial proteins. Analysis of gingival crevicular fluid (GCF) has been used for over 50 years as a non-invasive method of monitoring for infection below the gum line

The concentrations of the toxic thiols *hydrogen sulfide* and *methyl mercaptan sulfide* in GCF have been shown to positively correlate with the clinical measures of periodontal disease severity.(5)

Another aspect of periodontal testing that is extremely important is the fact that periodontal pockets can be "disease-active" or "disease-inactive." Traditional diagnostic procedures do not identify susceptible individuals nor distinguish between disease-active and disease-inactive periodontal sites.(6) *TOPAS* solves this problem because it is a true activity based assay. Only the presence of actively growing and dividing anaerobic pathogens will result in increased levels of these toxic metabolites: "Although pathogenic bacteria are often associated with disease, and often increase numerically during disease progression, the organisms are also often present in health and in non-progressing sites."(7) The mere presence of known or putative pathogens does not result in a positive *TOPAS* reaction.

DISCLAIMER: Although we are providing information related to a specific company and their particular tests, we are merely providing a source of information. Their inclusion in this book does not constitute

Oral Health and Heart Disease

an endorsement by the authors or Bio-Probe, Inc. Dentists and physicians who wish to investigate further, should visit their web site at http://www.altcorp.com. The same is true for patients desiring further information. The site provides a wide range of excellent information on mercury, autism and thimerosal, root canal toxicity as well as oral health diseases.

Diet:

Because we are proceeding on the basis of an anti-infective therapy, it is a logical extension to evaluate how diet might be impacting your immune systems ability to control putative pathogens involved in development of periodontal disease. Consequently, the BPT team is going to evaluate what foods you might be eating routinely, or excessively, that are bacteria friendly rather than immune system friendly. Dietary carbohydrates are a major source of energy for plaque bacteria, not only during chewing but also as food debris that remains in the mouth. Sucrose (common table sugar), normally found in manufactured foods, especially in confectionary products, plays a key role in plaque growth and in the development of caries. When certain plaque bacteria metabolize the sugar they also produce acid and fermentation of dietary carbohydrates by plaque also bring about an increase in acidity, which is what starts eating into the enamel and ultimately cause caries. The plaque and the acid environment also initiates inflammation of the gingiva. Consequently, if you are a heavy carbohydrate eater, dietary counseling and modification is a must if you are going to eliminate periodontal pathogens.

As we have stated previously, if your immune system is not functioning properly a nutritional assessment will help provide guidance as to which nutrients are needed to help overcome the immune deficiency. This may require some specific testing or diet evaluation to identify probable vitamin and mineral deficiencies and make specific recommendations if required.

Oral Health and Heart Disease

Medical Health Evaluation:

There are health conditions which the patient may not even be aware of. For instance diabetes can affect your ability to resist the invasion of periodontal pathogens. If your dentist suspects that or other health conditions which you have not indicated on your medical history he or she may require you take blood tests or other systemic tests to determine if any underlying problems do exist.

Treatment:

This will vary somewhat between dentists but the objectives remain the same. Disinfect the mouth and eliminate periodontopathic microorganisms while progressing slowly with any operative procedures that might require removal of tissue; remove calculus deposits; insure that the patient fully understands and is practicing proper oral hygiene and plaque control and fully understands the role of diet and good nutrition as well as the damage that can accrue from use of tobacco, alcohol and excessive use of refined sugars.

Subsequent appointments will evaluate compliance with home care procedures and protocols; supra and subgingival irrigation with antimicrobial agents; ultrasonic scaling and further manual calculus debridement as needed. If microbial cultures were taken originally, the possible application of antibiotic therapy, if warranted.

Follow-ups continue on a 3 month basis for moderate and higher levels of periodontal involvement until visual, microscopic or laboratory analysis indicates the original objectives are being achieved. When patient response and healing is slower, you may be required to be seen and treated every two months. Once objectives have been obtained and maintained through three or four appointments, scheduling may go to an annual treatment and evaluation.

We hope that after reading this book, you will have a better appreciation about the seriousness and complexity of periodontal disease and how very important it is to your health to treat your oral health as an essential requisite contributing to your overall longevity and well-being.

REFERENCES

1. Loesche WJ. The antimicrobial treatment of periodontal disease. Crit Rev Oral Biol Med 1999;10(3):245-275.

2. Corbet EE, Vaughan AJ and Kieser JB. The periodontally-involved root surface. J Clin Periodontol 1993;20:402-410.

3. Dahlen G., et al. The effect of supragingival plaque control on the subgingival microbiota in subjects with periodontal disease. J Clin Periodontol 1992;19:802-809.

4. Lamster IB. Evaluation of components of gingival crevicular fluid as diagnostic tests. Ann Periodontol 1997;2:123-137.

5. Persson S. Hydrogen sulfide and methyl mercaptain in periodontal pockets. Oral Microbiol Immunol 1992 Dec;7(6):378-379.

6. Page RC. Host response tests for diagnosing periodontal diseases. Periodontol 1992;63:365-366.

7. Williams RC, Beck JD, Offenbacher SN. The impact of new technologies to diagnose and treat periodontal disease. A look to the future. J Clin Periodontol 1996;23:299-305.

Oral Health and Heart Disease

Index

A

acetylcholine	
blocked by mercury	36
Acrodynia	
caused by mercury	32
acute myocardial infarction	
patients deficient in magnesium	63
acute myocardial infarction (AMI)	
periodontal disease	15
allergic reaction	
mercury	8
amalgam dental fillings	
chest pains, tachycardia, anemia, fatigue	28
contain 50% mercury	8
periodontal disease	9
American Academy of Periodontalogy	14
aspirating pheumonia	
periodontal disease	20
atheroclerotic plaques	
periodontal pathogens	15

B

bacteremia	
causes of	15
definition of	15
root canals	16
stroke and myocardial infarction	15
beri-beri	
caused by deficiency of thiamine	68
Betadine	
kills oral bacteria and viruses	48
Biocompatible Periodontal therapy (BPT)	75
biocompatible periodontal therapy	
definition of	75
diagnostic component	78
dietary considerations	80
medical health evaluation	80
treatment regimen	81
bone loss	
caused by magnesium deficiency in rats	60

C

calcium in heart muscle	
displaced by mercury	34
calculus	
definition of	61
cardiovascular disease	
magnesium can correct mitral valve prolapse	62
magnesium reduces incidence of arrhythmia	62
No. 1 cause of death	7
treatment with CoQ10	58
vitamin E reduces risk	65
Center for Disease Control	
fluorides action topical not systemic	47
cerebrovascular accidents (CVA)	
periodontal disease a risk factor	14
CoQ10	
coenzyme Q10	57
efficacy demonstrated in 8 year heart study	59
frequently deficient in gingivitis	57
gingival crevicular fluid flow	57
heart failure patients have lower levels	59
leucocyte CoQ10 deficient in periodontitis	57
topical application to treat gingivitis	57
use in cardiovascular disease	58
coronary artery disease	
vitamin E reduces risk	65
Coronary Heart Disease	
leading cause of death in the U.S.	7
Coronary Heart Disease (CHD)	
460,000 deaths annually	7

D

dental amalgam mercury vapor	
accumulates more rapidly in heart than brain	27
dental amalgam mercury	
accumulation in body tissues	25
high levels in pituitary of dentists	25
dental amalgam mercury vapor	
in animals accumulate in heart	26
dental caries	14

Oral Health and Heart Disease

can be caused by thiamine deficiency 68
dental mercury
    affects transsulfuration pathway 64
    binds to sulfur molecules 63
    can cause inflammation and periodontitis 63
    can increase homocysteine levels 64
    reduces metabolism of methionine 64
dental pain
    controlled by vitamin B1 and B6 70
    treatment with thiamine 68
diabetes
    periodontal disease 19

E

endodontic treatment
    can cause bacteremia 16

F

factor F
    ox-bile 45
fluoride information
    http://www.fluoridealert.org 47
folic acid 65
    critical to reduction of homocysteine 66
    deficiencies wide spread 66
    gingivitis one of the deficiency symptoms 66
FoliCare mouthwash
    1% folic acid solution 49
frusemide
    induces deficiency of thiamine 67

G

gingival crevicular fluid
    TOPAS test 79
gingival crevicular fluid (GCF)
    CoQ10 57
    definition of 78
grapefruit seed extract
    antimicrobial 49

H

heart failure
    treatment with thiamine corrected problem 68
herbal tooth pastes 47
herpes simplex
    treated with oral vitamin B1 69
herpes zoster
    treated with oral vitamin B1 69
hypertension
    mercury 32
hypoglycemia
    can effect periodontal tissue 20

I

idiopathic dilated cardiomyopathy
    greatly increased mercury levels in heart 25
infective endocarditis 14

K

Keyes Technique
    definition of 77
kidney stones
    magnesium inhibits formation of 61

L

low birth weight
    and periodontal disease 19
lung function
    diminishes with periodontal disease 21

M

magnesium 59
    daily intake deficit of 200 mg 60
    deficiency and acute myocardial infarction 63
    deficiency caused bone loss in rats 60
    half stored in soft tissue and half in bone 62
    inhibits formation of kidney stones 61
    involved in over 300 different enzyme systems 60
    less than 1% present in blood 62

Oral Health and Heart Disease

serum levels increased with vitamin B6   61
mercury
  Acrodynia   32
  affects hormones that regulate heart   37
  and your heart   23
  blocks the neurotransmitter acetylcholine   36
  damage to heart and blood vessels   31
  displaced calcium in heart muscle   34
  diuretics   23
  hypertension and tachycardia   32
  impaired cardiac electrical function   34
  increases blood coagulation   38
  levels in heart increase with age   24
  non-dental in cardiovascular tissues   23
  pathological damage to heart tissue   34
mercury diuretics
  treatment for congestive heart failure   23
mercury vapor
  increases exposure to heart   23
  passes the placenta and accumulates
    in fetus   39
mercury vapor exposure
  chest pains   36
  heart palpitations   36
  high blood pressure   36
  in animals caused abnormal ECG   36
  in animals caused slow heart beat   36
  irregular pulse   36
  rapid heart beat   36
metabolic acidosis
  corrected with thiamine   68
metastasis
  definition of   13
MistORAL
  oral mouth spray for gingivitis   49
mitral valve prolapse
  oral magnesium supplementation helped   62

N

NHANES III
  chronic obstructive pulmonary disease   20
nonsurgical periodontal treatment
  definition of   75

O

occlusion
  progression of periodontitis   17
oral irrigators
  Waterpik, Hydro Floss, Via-Jet   50
ox-bile
  to control calculus build-up   45

P

pain reduction   70
  vitamin C   70
  vitamin B1   70
  vitamin B6   70
  vitamin B12   70
  vitamin K   70
painful menstruation
  cured with oral vitamin B1   70
periodontal disease
  acute myocardial infarction   15
  aspirating pheumonia   20
  deficiency of CoQ10   57
  definition of   13
  diabetes   19
  effects of dental mercury   63
  heart disease   14
  hyperesthesia and low magnesium   60
  preterm low birth weight   19
  risk factor for stroke   14
  systemic diseases   19
  warning signs of   14
periodontal pathogens
  laboratory diagnosis of   78
personal hygiene
  antiseptics and antimicrobials   48
  Betadine antiseptic   48
  brushing your teeth   43
  FoliCare mouthwash   49
  grapefruit seed extract   49
  herbal toothpastes available   47
  MistORAL topical mouth spray   49
  mouthwash and irrigants   48
  oral irrigators   50
  propolis extract   49
  selection of proper toothpaste   47
  use of power toothbrushes   43

Oral Health and Heart Disease

Pharmaden
  periodontal nutritional formulas   71
  phase contrast microscope
    its use in BPT   78
Pima Indians
  non-insulin diabetes   20
plaque
  bacteria in plaque produce toxins   13
  reduced by tooth brushing   44
  power toothbrush
    reduce pain in dentin hypersensitivity   43
    reduce plaque and pain   43
  propolis extract
    antibacterial   49

R

risk factors for heart diease
  physical inactivity   7
  stress   7
risk factors for heart disease
  cigarette smoking   7
  diabetes   7
  high blood cholesterol levels   7
  high blood pressure   7
  obesity   7
root planing
  definition of   75

S

stroke
  will become leading cause of death   16
surgical periodontal treatment   75
Systemic Diseases
  related to periodontal disease   19

T

tachycardia
  mercury   32

thaimine (vitamin B1)
  required for metabolism of carbohydrates   66
  oral vitamin B1 cured painful
    menstruation   70
  reduced by diuretics   67
thiamine (vitamin B1)   66
  deficiency can cause acid saliva   68
  deficiency can lead to cardiac failure   67
  does dental mercury complex with
    thiamine   67
  helps CHF patients taking frusemide   67
  one of two vitamiins with sulfur
    molecules   67
  reduced by use of antibiotics   67
  treatment of dental pain   68
  reduced by high carbohydrate
    meals/snacks   67
The specific plaque hypothesis   75

V

vitamin C   55
  deficiency causes scurvy   56
  deficiency increases risk of stroke   56
  deficiency makes gums bleed easily   56
  deficiency reduces collagen formation   56
  improves vasomotor function   56
  reduces pain   70
vitamin E
  antioxidant   64
  decreased healing time after
    gingivectomy   65
  reduced alveolar bone loss in rats   65
  reduces risk of coronary heart disease   65
vitamin B6   70
  reduces pain   70
  involved in trytophan, serotonin, and
    dopamine metabolism   70
vitamin B12   70
  reduces pain   70